Don Green

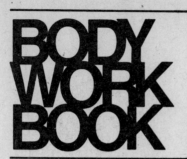

BODY WORK BOOK

BODY WORK BOOK

HERBERT HAESSLER, M.D.
AND
RAYMOND HARRIS

 AVON
PUBLISHERS OF BARD, CAMELOT AND DISCUS BOOKS

CREDITS AND ACKNOWLEDGMENTS

We acknowledge with thanks the help extended by the following individuals and organizations:

The New York Institute for Child Development for the use of their "Learning Disabilities Checklist."

Jack H. Hall, M.D. and Health Care Services, Inc., Methodist Hospital, Indianapolis, Indiana, for the use of information from Lewis C. Robbins and Jack H. Hall's *How to Practice Prospective Medicine*, 1970, and from *The Probability of Dying in the Next Ten Years from Specific Causes,* by Harvey Geller and Gregory Steele.

The Welch Allyn Company of Skaneateles Falls, N.Y. for pictures of medical equipment.

Medical Center Surgical Supply for illustrations and for information about the availability of medical equipment.

John V. Basmajian, M.D. and the Williams and Wilkins Company for the following anatomical drawings originally used in *Primary Anatomy,* seventh edition, 1976: paired palatine tonsils, female breast, villi of the small intestine, lymph nodes and drainage of the neck, muscles of the back.

Appleton-Century-Crofts for the following anatomical drawings from Helen L. Dawson's *Basic Human Anatomy,* second edition, 1974: the human skeleton, the vertebral column, a typical thoracic vertebra, upper arm muscles, muscles of the arm and hand, knee joint, the heart and its major blood vessels, the central nervous system, the cerebral hemispheres of the brain, sagittal section through the brain, the digestive system, sagittal section of the pharynx, the ear, structures of the skin, position of internal urinary organs, male reproductive organs, internal female reproductive organs, external female genitals.

Medequip Company of Rockville, MD. for information used in the systems review.

Christine Powers for expert research and editing, for sharing in the writing, and for assuming the awesome responsibility of creating a manuscript in its final form.

H.H. and R.H.

INTRODUCTION

There is a quiet revolution underway in medicine that promises to be as important in the prevention and treatment of disease and in prolonging life as the discovery of the "wonder drugs" was forty years ago.

For years it has seemed that the least important element in the treatment of disease and the maintenance of health was the patient. As medicine became more and more specialized, an illness became a bladder that responded to a sulfa drug—or it didn't. It was a chronic headache that responded to analgesics and tranquilizers—or it didn't. It was a joint or a circulatory system or a third lumbar vertebra, and they were all expected to act much the same way and could be treated according to norms, averages and percentages. And there was standard advice: "Let's not overdo and tax the old back. We're not as young as we used to be, you know." This last was usually said with the patronizing air of a doctor-father who knows everything to his patient-child who knows nothing, even though the patient may have been looking after his health and the health of his family with remarkable success for twenty years.

But with the recent resurgence of the general practice—now called family medicine—there is a renewed interest in the whole patient. Doctors now want to know how your whole body is functioning in the particular environment in which you live. There is more interest in what you do to your body and how your body functions in the conduct of your everyday life. And doctors have come to realize that there is no one better able to furnish this information than the owner of the body.

Everyone has certain expertise about his own body which, until now, has gone unrecognized and unused, for the most part, in the diagnosis and treatment of disease. Consequently, the revolution in medicine is aimed at establishing a continuous doctor-patient partnership where the patient monitors the functioning of his or her body under all sorts of circumstances and situations.

In this sort of partnership you become what is being called an educated or "activated" patient. You take an active interest in your body, its parts, and how it works as an integrated whole. You come to know what looks and feels normal for you (normal is not the same for everyone), and to know what is not normal that requires the attention of your physician. Then, when you report to your partner, the doctor, either for a checkup or because of illness, you can give him or her an intelligent and knowledgeable appraisal of what's going on. And best of all, you talk to one another on an equal plane about a common problem you are trying to solve together. Gone is the Herr Doktor who dominates a silent and submissive patient.

More attention is being paid to teaching people health-producing behavior. In the new relationship, the individual has a certain responsibility for his own health, and you and your physician educate each other in the special intricacies of the only body in the world that is exactly like yours.

Your medical history is the most important diagnostic instrument available to your doctor. Studies have shown that 85 percent of the time, a correct diagnosis of what ails you is made on the basis of medical history alone. And the more you know about yourself from constant observation and monitoring, the more you are able to tell the doctor. What is more, a close look at your medical history and your life style (both of which are more complete under your own scrutiny than under your doctor's) can tell you, statistically, what your chances are for surviving the next ten years and what you can do to develop a survival advantage—that is, what you can do to add years to your life beyond your present prospects. We will show you how to do this.

While examinations and tests in the doctor's office are important, there are some very important questions they can't answer.

- What pulse rate is normal for you under a variety of circumstances—at work, play, and rest?
- What is your blood pressure when you are not experiencing the stress of a visit to the doctor? How does it vary from day to day?
- How quickly does your breathing and heartbeat return to normal after stress?
- Is 98.6° F. a "normal" temperature for you? (Some people are normal at 97, others at 99 degrees.)

You can do many tests yourself, at home, and under the new doctor-patient partnership your doctor will not only want you to do them, he will expect it of you.

Oral and rectal thermometers have been familiar diagnostic tools in many homes for years. If you have not yet learned to use them, you should do so as soon as possible. When you call the doctor's office about a sick child, the first thing you will be asked is, "Does the child have a fever?" You will be expected to know.

There is nothing mysterious about taking a pulse. You should know where your pressure points are and what the normal ranges of the pulse beat are for you and other members of the family. You should be able to tell what a strong, regular pulse feels like. Even a flashlight is an important diagnostic instrument once you know what to do with it. No doctor is ever without a penlight in his pocket, and you should never be without one either.

You can also check your own blood pressure. The impressive sounding *sphygmomanometer* (for testing blood pressure) is now available for under $50 and is easy to use. The stethoscope—that ultimate sign of doctorhood—can be had in cheap throwaway models. While they are not like your doctor's sophisticated instrument and might not pick up an elusive murmur, they can still provide valuable information about the sounds made by your heart and lungs.

Some examinations you do yourself can save your life. Most breast cancers in their early stages (when they are most treatable) are discovered by women testing themselves. Melanoma, a particularly vicious and invasive form of skin cancer when it is allowed to get a start on you, is best caught in its earliest stages by an alert person who keeps track of skin blemishes. Slight bleeding somewhere in the digestive tract can be detected, before it can be seen in the stools, with a simple test available in the drugstore.

An alert home examiner can discover early signs of scoliosis in a young person, a spinal curvature that must be spotted early for successful treatment. Early discovery of sugar or other substances in the urine, using tests available in the drugstore, warns you to see your doctor at once before a potential problem becomes serious and more difficult to treat. By tracking your vision, you may discover subtle changes in the way you see that signal serious trouble and possible blindness which can be avoided with prompt medical attention.

Much of the mystery is going out of medical examinations and most doctors are glad to see it go. It is being replaced by the intelligence, awareness, and common sense of informed patients who know their own bodies because they feel, see, and hear what is going on with that marvelous machine on a day-to-day, continuing basis. This is the revolution in medicine that will provide longer, healthier lives for millions of people. It is hoped that this book will help to make you a part of the revolution and such a devotee of the cause that you will carry the word to others.

TABLE OF CONTENTS

BODY
WORK
BOOK

CHAPTER 1

TESTING THE HEART, LUNGS, AND CIRCULATION

The heart is the traditional center of life, love, courage, and all of our best and worst emotions. I give you my heart when I'm in love, I have a stout heart when I'm brave, a true heart when I'm faithful, I'm bighearted when I'm kind and generous, blackhearted when I'm a dastardly knave, fainthearted when I'm cowardly, and downhearted when I'm blue. Couple this with the fact that more people die from heart and circulatory disease and malfunction than from any other cause, and it's no wonder that people worry more about their hearts than about any other part of the body.

Worry, however, doesn't do your heart a bit of good. Anxiety about the heart can, and often does, cause needless incapacity in people who are actually well. What is better than worrying is getting to know your heart and treating it like the sturdy (should we say stouthearted?) friend that it is.

The heart is a pump which moves blood throughout your entire body. Blood carries not only oxygen but all essential nutrients to every organ, every muscle, every bone, every cell. It also carries waste products away from the cells that comprise body tissues. If they have no blood moving through them, many tissues die rather quickly. If the flow of blood is interrupted to the brain for any reason, irreversible damage occurs after five minutes.

So the heart is a very important organ. It is also a very well-designed and dependable organ that pumps along consistently, about 72 times a minute, 100,000 times a day, moving about 2,000 gallons of blood without your being aware of it for the most part. And that's the way it should be. It will get along very nicely by itself without your worrying about it.

GETTING TO KNOW YOUR HEART

The heart is a very muscular organ. It is divided in half by a wall or septum which runs through the middle of the heart, inside, from top to bottom. Each side has two chambers, making four chambers in all—two auricles or atria that receive blood, and two ventricles that pump it out again.

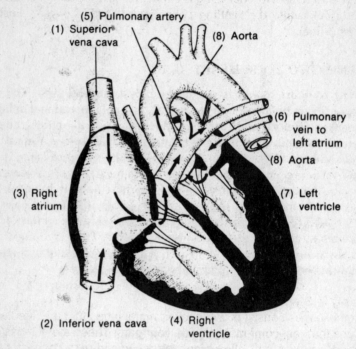

Diagram of the Heart

(1) Superior vena cava from upper body; (2) inferior vena cava from lower body; (3) right atrium of the heart; (4) right ventricle of the heart; (5) pulmonary artery to the lungs; (6) pulmonary vein returns blood from the lungs to the left atrium of the heart; (7) left ventricle of the heart; (8) aorta carries blood to the body.

A highly efficient system of valves keeps blood flowing in the right direction, a rich network of blood vessels keeps the heart supplied with oxygen while it works, and a built-in pacemaker keeps the pumping action going at a regular rate. An automatic control system regulates the speed and strength of the pumping action in response to a complicated set of signals from various parts of the body. It all works so well that it couldn't be better if you had designed it yourself.

The two sides of the heart work in unison. The right side pumps blood through the lungs to collect oxygen. The oxygen-rich blood then returns to the left side of the heart and from there it is pumped to the rest of the body. The heart pumps blood by alternately squeezing to force blood into the blood vessels and then relaxing to allow the chambers to refill. The squeezing is called the systolic action or systole (sis'-tuh-lee), while the refilling phase is called diastolic or diastole (di-aś-tuh-lee).

LISTENING TO YOUR HEART

Listening to heart sounds is one of the oldest medical tests. You can hear your heart beating quite easily with a simple instrument called a stethoscope. Before stethoscopes, doctors used a hollow tube to amplify the sound, and before that they just laid an ear against the patient's chest which, in some cases, was the fun way of doing it.

Until rather recently, a stethoscope was a mysterious instrument to be used by doctors only. Left hanging around the neck, it distinguished the doctors from the rest of the staff in a hospital. Stethoscopes became popular for home use once we began to realize the importance of individuals monitoring their own blood pressure. They are now widely available at medical supply stores, at some drugstores, or sometimes through advertisements in newspapers and magazines.

Using a Stethoscope

All stethoscopes consist of two hooked metal tubes that are fitted with earplugs that rest comfortably inside your ears. These metal tubes are attached to rubber or plastic tubing which is joined by a connector and then continues into a single tube which ends in either a flat or bell-shaped piece that is placed against the patient's chest to pick up sound.

Look at the ear pieces of your stethoscope. Notice that the ear plugs have a slant to them. Hold the stethoscope in front of you turned so that the curve or slant of the earplugs points slightly forward, away from you. Now place one of the ear plugs in each ear.

To listen to your heart, place the flat or bell-shaped chest piece against your chest a little below the left nipple and just a bit toward the middle of your chest. Women should place the chest piece as close to the inside margin of the breast as possible. In order to hear your heart well you must have good contact between your chest wall and the chest

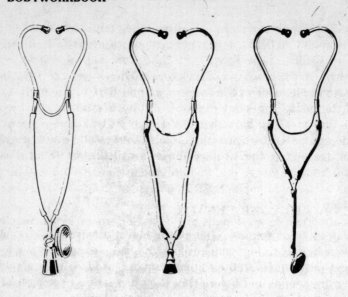

Stethoscopes

piece of the stethoscope. If the chest piece is rocking on a rib, move it slightly until it lies completely flat and firm against your skin.

Listen carefully and you will hear your heart beating. It beats a little more often than once each second, about 72 times per minute. Each beat consists of two sounds which quickly follow each other. You should hear something which sounds like lub-dub, lub-dub. Move your stethoscope around a bit until the beat is loudest. The heart sounds will be slightly different in different parts of your chest. You should be able to hear your heart sounds from just below the inner edge of your collar bone on the left down to just above the next to last rib. You will usually be able to hear your heart more clearly near the central part of your chest than way out at the side.

Some people's heart sounds are much more easily heard than others. It is relatively easy to hear heart sounds in people with thin chest walls, and it is much more difficult to hear chest sounds in fat people. However, except under unusual circumstances, difficulty in hearing heart sounds is not an indication of disease. If you have trouble finding an area where you can hear your heart sounds clearly, put your whole open hand over the lower part of your chest just under the left nipple. Sit up and lean forward. You should be able to feel your heart beating. The place where the heartbeat feels strongest is called the point of maximum impulse. Put the chest piece of the stethoscope here.

After you have found the various areas where you can hear your heart beating, listen carefully to the sounds. The two sounds come fairly close together: lub-dub, lub-dub. There should be a short space between the pairs of sounds where you hear little if anything. The heart should beat regularly, anywhere from about 60 to 80 times each minute. If you are an athlete or participate in an exercise program, your heart rate may be just a little under 60 beats per minute. And as you have surely noticed long before this, your heart beats faster when you exercise or if you are nervous.

Most abnormal heart sounds are called murmurs. A murmur is a sort of blowing sound and occurs most frequently between the two major heart sounds—that is, between the lub and the dub. If you have a heart murmur it may sound like lub-shsss-dub, lub-shsss-dub. But sometimes murmurs occur after the end of the second heart sound, giving a lub-dub-shsss, lub-dub-shsss.

Many people who are perfectly well and healthfully active have heart murmurs, so if you find you have a heart murmur, *don't panic*. But go see your physician and have it checked.

The fact that you have a murmur does not mean that something dreadful is about to happen. Although murmurs are sometimes an indication of heart disease, many people who have serious heart disease do not have murmurs and many people who have murmurs actually have very little wrong with their hearts. In years gone by, many children were unncessarily restricted in their activities because "the doctor said they had a heart murmur," and frantic relatives treated the poor child as an invalid who was not long for this world. Today, a murmur is evaluated carefully by the doctor, and if the verdict is that it's nothing to worry about, then don't worry about it.

If you are listening to your heart—or especially if you are listening to a youngster's or an elderly person's heart—you might be startled to notice a rather marked change in the rate of the heartbeat. If you observe closely, this condition can often be related to breathing in and out. As a breath is drawn in, the heartbeat speeds up. Upon breathing out, the heartbeat slows down. Usually there are no signs of discomfort or distress associated with this condition and it is entirely harmless. It is something that characteristically appears in children, disappears in middle life, and then frequently reappears as one gets older.

You will rarely encounter other irregularities in the heartbeat while listening through a stethoscope in a person who is apparently well.

Certain severe irregularities occur in people who are desperately ill, but in such cases you won't need a stethoscope to know they are in trouble and in need of immediate medical attention.

But almost everyone *feels* an irregular heartbeat in themselves from time to time. You might feel your heart skip a beat, or it might seem to race or palpitate, causing some discomfort and worry. Sometimes this happens when you are nervous or after an evening of too much of everything—especially too much coffee, liquor, and cigarettes. More often than not, these irregularities are harmless if they don't persist, but because they are disturbing, it's a good idea to have a doctor check into it—if only for the sake of reassurance and to hear once again that you should quit smoking and come out from under your stressful life style.

FOR YOUR PERSONAL HEALTH RECORD

1. Listen carefully to your heart sounds. Describe what you hear as best you can.

2. On your next visit to your doctor describe your impressions of the sound—"It sounds good and strong," "It seems to speed up and slow down," or "I think I detect a murmur," and so on. Compare this with what your doctor says.

3. After visiting the doctor, listen again yourself. In a brief comment, record what the doctor has told you as compared with what you hear yourself.

CHECKING YOUR PULSE

Each time the heart beats there is a corresponding impulse in major blood vessels throughout the body. At points where arteries come near the surface of the body, these impulses can be felt quite easily. Since the impulses correspond exactly with your heartbeat, if you want to determine how fast your heart is beating it is easier to feel for the impulses than to listen to the heart. This is what you do when you check your *pulse*.

You can find a pulse beat just below your inside ankle bone, in your temples, on either side of your Adam's apple, and at several other places around the body. But the most popular and accessible place to take a pulse is on the wrist just below the base of the thumb.

Taking a Pulse

1. Turn one hand palm up and wrap the fingers of your other hand around the wrist from the back so that the tips of your fingers are touching the wrist where you are taking the pulse, just below the base of the thumb. Grasp the wrist firmly without squeezing. By grasping with all your fingers, you should feel the throbbing pulse beat at once. (DO NOT use your thumb. You can often feel a pulse in your thumb so that the pulse on pulse can be confusing, especially when you take the pulse of another person.) If you just poke at your wrist with one finger, you may have to move it around a bit before you find a spot where the pulse can be felt distinctly.

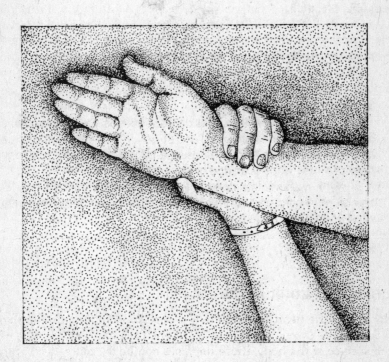

2. When you take someone else's pulse it will probably be easier for you if they turn their hand with the palm facing down, and then you can wrap your fingers around the top of their wrist, so that the tips of your fingers rest on the underside of their wrist at the base of the thumb.

3. Have a watch or a clock handy that has an easy-to-see sweep second hand. Make sure you can feel the beat of the pulse under your fingertips and as the second hand crosses a well-defined spot on the dial of the watch (12, 3, 6, and 9 are favorite positions), begin to count pulse beats.

4. Although you want the number of times the pulse beats in a minute, you do not have to wait a whole minute to get your results. If the pulse feels steady and regular, count for just 10 seconds and multiply by six. Or, count for 15 seconds and multiply by four.

If absolute accuracy is desired, as when you are recording for exercise and fitness charts, you might count as long as 30 seconds and multiply by two to reduce possible error. And here's a tip in pulse counting that more than 25 percent of doctors aren't aware of, as was found in a recent test: Make your first count *zero* as the second hand crosses the mark you have set—0, 1, 2, 3, etc. This is one of those obvious things that isn't obvious at all until you twist your thinker out of joint thinking about it.

Except for stress tests and measures of physical condition during exercise, the pulse should be measured at rest.

Many people have heard that a *normal* pulse rate when you are relaxed is 72 beats per minute. What is meant is that the *average* pulse rate of normally healthy people in our population is 72 beats per minute. Athletes, and people in very good physical condition who exercise regularly, will often have slow pulse rates, sometimes 60 or even lower when they are relaxed. Smokers and people in poor physical condition tend to have higher pulse rates.

Exercise, of course, increases the pulse rate. A young athlete in good condition can tolerate a peak performance pulse of 150 without difficulty. The pulse rate also increases with anxiety, emotional upset, excitement, and sexual activity.

Pulse rates of small children can be normal when more than 90 beats per minute. But pulse rates, at rest, that are above 80 may indicate a problem in adults. The pulse increases about 5 to 10 beats per minute for every degree of body temperature above what is normal for you. (98.6°F. is an *average* normal. Normal for you may be a little lower or a little higher.) So if your temperature is hovering around 101°F., your pulse rate may be as high as 92.

Severe anemia, thyroid disease, and some infections all increase the pulse rate. If your resting pulse rate is regularly over 80, or at the most 85 beats per minute, you should bring this to the attention of your doctor.

A slower than normal pulse rate can occur in a few acute illnesses, but these are also associated with other much more obvious physical discomforts that would prompt you to seek the help of a physician. More often, people with acute illnesses have abnormally fast pulse rates.

Someone who has had a sudden heart attack, who is going into shock for some reason, or has severe pain, will usually have a very fast pulse rate. In someone who is acutely ill the quality of the pulse is often poor. It is not only rapid but is sometimes described as "thin" or "thready." This means that the beats are not very strong. Anyone who seems acutely ill and has a fast, thready pulse rate needs immediate medical attention.

Since "normal" can vary so widely among people, it is a good idea to know what your resting, relaxed pulse is when you are well. Then you will be in a position to observe deviations from what is normal for you. If you are in a gradually increasing physical-conditioning program, if you have learned to be less anxious, if you have lost excess weight in a supervised weight loss program, or if you have given up smoking, excess alcohol, and coffee, chances are good you will notice a decline in your normal pulse rate. Generally speaking, if you are also feeling well, this is just what the doctor ordered.

If your resting pulse rate rises and stays appreciably above what you have established as normal for you, or if your pulse is "normally" over 80, you and your doctor should try to find out why.

Pulse Rate and the Step Test.   When you undertake a regular exercise program to improve the tone and fitness of your cardiovascular and pulmonary systems, you will find that your resting pulse rate gradually becomes lower and lower, and levels off as you approach peak fitness for you. It is not unusual, for instance, for a person to start with a pulse of 80 beats per minute and drop to 50 or 60 beats per minute after several months of regular exercise.

If you are in a program of regular exercise, you can track the improvement in your pulse rate by using the step test.

The Two-Minute Step Test
CAUTION: If in the course of this test you feel chest discomfort or pain, dizziness or uncomfortable fatigue, stop at once and consult a physician. The step test as described is equivalent to climbing six or seven flights of stairs at a fast pace. If you have been sedentary and are just beginning to exercise, if you have a heart problem, if you are recovering from an illness, or if you are over thirty-five and have not

been exercising regularly, do not try this test without first checking with a doctor.

1. Using a sturdy and stable bench or stool about 15 inches high, step up onto the stool so that you are standing on it with both feet. Then step down and stand on the floor again.

2. Repeat stepping on and off the stool this way for two minutes at the rate of thirty round trips a minute (onto and back off the stool once every two seconds). You may need a partner to time your movements and you will probably have to practice a bit to establish a smooth rhythm.

3. At the end of two minutes of exercise, sit down and rest for two minutes.

4. After resting for two minutes take your pulse. Record the result and try again in about two weeks. If you exercise regularly in the meantime, you should find your pulse gradually slowing down.

FOR YOUR PERSONAL HEALTH RECORD

1. Take a *resting* pulse rate several mornings in a row before you get out of bed. Record your *average* resting pulse rate on your health record.

2. Recheck every six months and record any changes. Record any changes in living habits that might affect the pulse—smoking, drinking, exercise patterns, stress, use of drugs, etc. Make any comments you feel are appropriate.

3. If you are in a supervised exercise program, track and record pulse changes in consultation with your doctor or athletic supervisor. If you are in a nonsupervised program, track your pulse every two weeks using the step test.

TAKING YOUR OWN BLOOD PRESSURE

High blood pressure, also known as hypertension, has been shown to be so closely related to the incidence of heart attacks and strokes that it is known, quite appropriately, as "the silent killer." At any one time, as many as 23 million people in the United States have abnormally high blood pressure—and most of them don't even know it.

In recent years, an all-out effort has been launched to convince people that it is important for them to monitor their blood pressure.

Blood-pressure clinics are conducted with increasing frequency where people work, as projects of civic organizations, in drugstores and supermarkets, or anyplace where large numbers of people can hear the word and be tested. It has become almost an evangelical movement.

Where taking blood pressure was once reserved for the hospital and the doctor's office, people are now encouraged to keep close tabs on their own blood pressure. To measure your blood pressure you need your stethoscope and a blood-pressure cuff whose official name is sphygmomanometer (sfig'-moh-muh-nom-i-ter). The name comes from the Greek word *sphygmus,* which is simply our old friend the pulse, and *meter* which means measure.

Blood-pressure cuffs are readily available from medical supply stores, from drugstores, and through mail-order advertisements in many popular magazines and catalogs. They have even found their way into the vending-machine trade, having been placed in shopping malls and department stores where you can take your own blood pressure for 50¢. Many instruments are now being designed to make them easier to use by yourself.

When your heart pumps, it pushes blood into the arteries throughout your body. As long as the heart keeps pumping, the flow of blood is continuous. The heart, however, pumps with an intermittent squeezing action. Each beat includes a squeeze which you can feel as a pulse. With each beat the blood pressure rises to a peak level, and between these it falls to a lower level. The highest level the blood pressure reaches is called the systolic pressure. This occurs when the heart is in systole, or when it is in its squeezing phase. The lowest level the blood pressure reaches is called the diastolic pressure. This occurs in diastole, or when the heart is refilling. Blood pressure is normally recorded as two numbers, such as 120 over 74 (120/74). The first, or larger, of the two numbers is the systolic pressure; the second, or smaller, is the diastolic pressure. The units of measurement of blood pressure are millimeters of mercury, the same units used to measure the atmospheric or barometric pressure recorded in weather reports. It is the amount of pressure necessary to hold up a column of mercury a certain number of millimeters high. Some blood-pressure recording machines actually use mercury columns for measurement, while others have a simple dial.

Increased interest in home testing has led to the development of new kinds of blood-pressure testing instruments, including one that provides an automatic digital read-out. Before you buy, make careful inquiries about guarantees of accuracy as you would when buying a camera, stereo components, or any other equipment and be sure you get a set of instructions. If in doubt, ask your doctor or other health professionals about their preferences. The use of dial or mercury-column types of sphygmomanometers are the ones most generally used at the moment, so these are the kinds we will talk about here.

Normal systolic pressures in adults range from about 110 to 145. Normal diastolic pressures range from about 60 to 90. In someone who seems well and is able to be up and about, low blood pressure has relatively little significance except that it is infinitely better to have low blood pressure than high blood pressure. High blood pressure—that is, pressure above 145 over 90—is a dangerous disorder.

Both exercise and emotional tension can elevate blood pressure. However, if your resting blood pressure is consistently above 145 over 90, you should consult your doctor promptly. It can't be emphasized too strongly that untreated high blood pressure is a dangerous disease which can eventually lead to a substantially shortened life because of either a heart attack or a stroke. And elevated blood pressure can be very effectively treated with several different medicines. It should be noted, too, that contrary to common belief, high blood pressure is not reserved exclusively for older people. It is not uncommon for some young people to have badly elevated blood pressure that should be treated as soon as it is discovered.

Measuring Blood Pressure

1. Wrap the blood-pressure cuff snugly around your upper arm, just above the elbow joint.

2. Tighten the thumb screw at the base of the inflation bulb. Inflate the cuff by pumping the bulb until the dial shows about 200 millimeters of mercury. This will give quite a hard squeeze on the upper arm.

3. Bend the arm just a little bit at the elbow and place either the bell or the diaphragm of the stethoscope in the little cupped part of the elbow joint.

4. Listen carefully with your stethoscope as you release the air pressure from the cuff. This is done by releasing the thumb screw that you tightened.

5. As the pressure comes down, you will suddenly begin to hear thumping sounds in your stethoscope. These will be regular and uniform sounds, one thump for each heart beat. Note the pressure at which you first begin to hear thumping sounds. This is the systolic pressure.

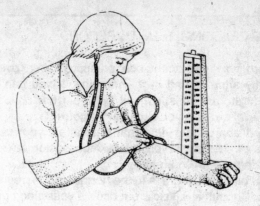

Using a Blood-pressure Cuff

6. Continue listening as you let pressure out of the cuff. Note the pressure at which you stop hearing thumping sounds. This is the diastolic pressure.

7. Reinflate the cuff and take the measurements several times to be sure you have done the test accurately.

Since many things can affect your blood pressure, it is a good idea to keep careful notes of the time of day when you do your test, your activity immediately preceding the test (include such things as arguments, worry, and other tension-causing situations). If you are taking any drug or medicine, record the fact and tell what it is. When you begin testing, take your blood pressure at least three days in a row under quiet, peaceful circumstances; shortly after you wake up in the morning is an ideal time.

If the results you get are inconsistent or confusing, bring your equipment to your doctor or another person who takes blood pressure frequently and professionally. Review your procedure and compare results with your equipment and with theirs. If there is a discrepancy in equipment, have it checked by your medical equipment dealer.

If you are under a doctor's care for hypertension, follow his or her directions explicitly. You may be directed to take your blood pressure under a variety of circumstances or before and after using your medication.

FOR YOUR PERSONAL HEALTH RECORD

1. Record your average blood pressure taken over several days, shortly after waking in the morning. If you can't get reasonably consistent results, consult with your doctor. Check your equipment and be sure you are using it correctly.

2. Record appropriate data that may affect your blood pressure: drugs or medicines you are taking, tension-causing situations, smoking or drinking, etc.

3. If your blood pressure is in the normal range, recheck every six months. Consult a physician at once if your blood pressure is higher than 145/90 for either the systolic or diastolic reading.

THE ELECTROCARDIOGRAM

The third basic technique used to study the heart function is the electrocardiogram. All muscles move in response to very small electric currents produced by nerve impulses. When these electric impulses are recorded from the heart muscle, the result is called an electrocardiogram.

The electrocardiogram is not a test you can do yourself, for two reasons: First, the testing machine—an electrocardiograph—is very expensive. Secondly, you would not be able to read the output of the machine without a considerable amount of special study and training.

An electrocardiogram of your heart's function, however, is an essential part of a complete physical checkup for adults, especially if you are approaching forty from either side, and you may be interested in looking at the results with your doctor.

The electrical action of your heart muscle is recorded by the electrocardiograph from various locations around your body, and a slightly different electrical tracing is recorded from each location. It is now standard procedure to record from twelve different locations. This is called the twelve-lead electrocardiogram. Each time your heart beats, the electrocardiograph records a series of waves. These have arbitrarily been named the P, Q, R, S, and T waves. The big up-and-down spike in the middle of each wave sequence is called the QRS complex. This represents the major mass of heart muscle contracting.

What might appear to be minor changes in the shapes of some of the waves are very important in the diagnosis of heart disease. For example, if the little flat segment between the end of the QRS complex

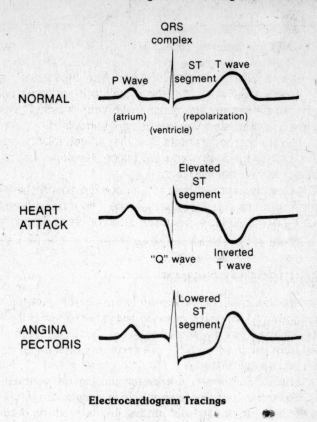

Electrocardiogram Tracings

and the low hump at the end, called the T wave, is either substantially depressed or elevated, it could mean that serious heart disease is present.

Tracking pulse rate, blood pressure, and making electrocardiogram tracings have assumed new importance in recent years as they are used in monitoring the progress of people engaged in physical-fitness and conditioning programs. If you have begun a fitness program—gym, jogging, walking, bicycling, lap swimming, or whatever—you should have a thorough medical evaluation at the outset to determine your capabilities, and then plan some way with your doctor or coach to monitor your progress.

Special programs have been developed for high-risk individuals and even for those who have suffered heart attacks. The results, whether a person starts out in the best or worst physical condition, have been uniformly good. And when you know how to monitor your own vital signs, it is most encouraging to watch your heart and pulse rates slow down and your blood pressure drop as your body responds to regular conditioning.

FOR YOUR PERSONAL HEALTH RECORD

1. Consult your doctor about the condition of your cardiovascular system. Include an electrocardiogram.
2. Discuss the results with your doctor (ask to see the tape tracing of the electrocardiogram and have it explained). Record the date and the doctor's findings in your health record.
3. Record dates and results of all future tests and discuss any differences or changes with the doctor.

RESPIRATORY RATE, LUNG CAPACITY, AND THE SOUNDS OF BREATHING

The main function of the lungs is to provide oxygen for the entire body and to get rid of the waste gas we produce in respiration—carbon dioxide. Respiration is the process in which body cells take in oxygen which is carried to them by the blood and give up waste carbon dioxide which is formed as the cells produce energy and go about the business of their highly specialized functions. The waste carbon dioxide is carried to the lungs by the blood where it is disposed of as you breathe out. The blood picks up fresh oxygen from air breathed in by the lungs and makes its next delivery to the cells. And so it goes for as long as you live.

When the body is called upon to work harder, as happens when you exercise, a complicated set of signals starts the heart pumping faster and the lungs breathing faster in order to fulfill the demand from the cells for more oxygen. If, for some reason, either your heart or lungs can't keep pace with the demand, you will find your ability to exercise, climb stairs, or run for a bus severely limited.

One of the fundamental measures of bodily function is the respiratory rate. This is the number of times you breathe in and out in one minute. A normal rate varies between fourteen and twenty times per minute. As with the heart rate, both exercise and fever raise the respiratory rate. A disorder of your thyroid gland may also increase your respiratory rate a little. Fever increases the respiratory rate about four breaths per minute for *every degree of fever above* **98.6° F.**

It is difficult to count your own respiratory rate because you become self-conscious and tend to breathe either faster or slower than you might when you are not paying attention to it. That's why a nurse will probably watch your respiratory rate while you think she is still check- ing your pulse. But with a little practice you should be able to count your respiratory rate without altering it because of self-consciousness. If not, ask someone else to catch you unawares and report it for you.

You can learn the way your lungs sound as they breathe in and out in the same way you learned how the heart sounds, by listening to them.

Listening to Your Breath Sounds

1. Place your stethoscope earplugs in your ears and place the chest piece firmly against your chest. Start on the right side of your chest, just below the nipple. Women should start just below the right breast.

2. Open your mouth and take a deep breath. Then blow the breath out slowly.

3. Breathe in and out slowly with your mouth open. You should be able to hear very soft breath sounds in and out each time you breathe. Normal breath sounds sound about the way your breath sounds after you have been running and are breathing hard.

4. Move the stethoscope around to various areas of your chest—up high, down low, around the sides, and around the back. You will notice that your doctor does most of his listening to your lungs from the back. This is partly because the breath sounds are a bit louder from the back and partly because the heartbeat is not as loud in the back, making it easier to hear the sounds in the left lung. You will not be able to reach very much of your own back with a stethoscope, but go back as far as you can, or work with a partner.

If you have asthma you may hear some abnormal breath sounds like little squeaks and whistles. During an asthma attack these squeaks and whistles become very apparent; but even when the asthma is not giving any trouble there are usually a few squeaks and whistles anyway, which, in an asthmatic person, have little meaning.

When you have a cold you may also hear some abnormal breath sounds. These are caused by mucous in the upper airways and gener- ally have little significance. Heavy smokers may also have some strange sounds caused by mucous accumulation.

A third kind of sound you may hear when you are sick is a very fine crackling sound. This is not very loud and sounds a bit like tissue paper being crumpled up. These are called rales and are usually heard when serious illness is present. Any abnormal collection of fluid in the lungs may cause rales. Pneumonia causes rales and lung congestion from heart failure also causes rales. Naturally, in such situations, immediate medical attention is indicated and many other signs of distress will be obvious.

Absolutely normal breath sounds are just the smooth flow of air in and out. If you hear other sounds and you are not sure what they are, it is best to ask your doctor.

Another instrument which your doctor may use in testing your lungs is a spirometer. This is an instrument which measures the amount of air that your lungs can hold. The doctor will either tell you to hold your nose or will give you a nose clip to wear. Then, he will ask you to take as deep a breath as possible, put your mouth over the spirometer tube, and blow all the air out as far as possible. The spirometer will then tell the doctor what the volume of air is that you can take into and expel from your lungs. This is called the vital capacity. Normal vital capacity varies tremendously with age, sex, and body size, but the normal range runs from about 3 to 6 liters. (A liter is just a little over a quart.)

The spirometer is a delicately balanced instrument and can be used for timing the speed with which you can move air out of your lungs, as well as measuring vital capacity. Like the cardiograph, it is not an instrument that is practical for you to own. But it is possible for you to find out if your vital capacity is relatively satisfactory without using a spirometer.

Testing Vital Capacity

1. Obtain the following items: a length of garden hose about three feet long, a tub like a large dishpan, and a bottle of at least a gallon capacity and not larger than two gallons.

2. Fill the bottle with water and fill the dishpan about half full with water.

3. Holding your hand over the mouth of the bottle, invert it in the dishpan so that the top of the bottle is under water. Have someone hold the bottle so it doesn't fall over, or prop it up in the dishpan. Be sure that the top of the bottle is not resting on the bottom of the dishpan.

4. Insert one end of the garden hose two to three inches up into the neck of the bottle without losing any of the water from the bottle. You won't lose any water as long as you keep the neck of the bottle submerged.

5. Hold your nose, take as deep a breath as you can and blow it all

into the garden hose. This will displace the water from the bottle and leave it partially filled with air.

6. Make a mark on the side of the bottle to show how much air you have blown into it.

7. Empty the bottle, stand it right side up and fill it with water up to your mark. The amount of water it takes to fill the bottle to the mark is the amount of air you were able to blow into the bottle.

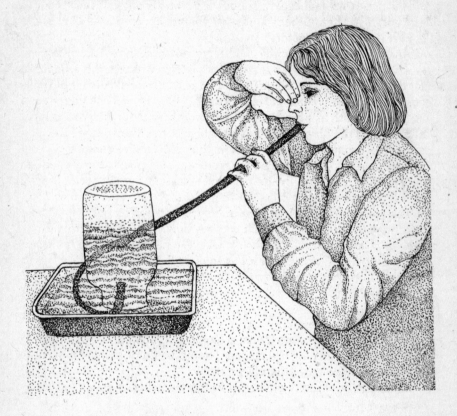

Since there is a rather high back pressure in this water system, you will probably not reach the vital capacity that you can on a doctor's spirometer. But if you can do better than half empty a gallon bottle (something over two quarts), your vital capacity will be at least average. If you can blow all the water out of a gallon bottle this way, you have quite a set of bellows. You will find that large people have greater vital capacities than smaller people and that in general smokers have smaller vital capacities than nonsmokers of the same body size.

A change in vital capacity over a period of time is more significant than a single measurement, so this is something you might want to do every six months or so. If you have breathing difficulties associated with vital capacity that declines over a period of time, you should definitely call it to the attention of your doctor.

Heavy smokers in their middle years who are also rather sedentary in their life style are likely to notice a marked decline in their vital capacity from year to year. So the water test or a spirometer test can sometimes be used as a potent argument against smoking and in favor of more exercise.

Even more important than the vital capacity is a test called the one-second forced expiratory volume. This is the total amount of air you can blow out after you have taken a deep breath and you blow out as hard as you can and as fast as you can. Although it is not possible to perform this test without a spirometer, there is a very simple test you can do to see whether you fall into the normal range.

Match Test

Light an ordinary paper match and hold it at arm's length. Then take a deep breath and try to blow the match out. You must aim straight, of course, but if you can blow the match out, your one-second forced expiratory volume is probably normal. This is a fairly sensitive test of lung function, so if you find you cannot move enough air to blow out a match at arm's length, consult your doctor because you may be developing lung disease that should be treated.

FOR YOUR PERSONAL HEALTH RECORD

1. Record your respiratory rate while at rest. Recheck every six months.

2. Describe any breathing sounds you hear other than a smooth flow of air.

3. Record vital capacity from a spirometer test or from the water bottle test. Recheck every six months. If you smoke, check every two or three months. A decline in vital capacity should be discussed with your physician.

4. Record pass or fail on the forced expiratory volume (match) test.

CHAPTER 2

TESTING VISION

In the days before television, the way the eyes work was best described in terms of the famous Brownie box camera, and as far as it goes, the analogy is still a good one. Both eye and camera are enclosed receptacles with a small hole in front to admit light rays. Both have a diaphragm to regulate the amount of light entering the optical system and both have a lens that focuses the light on a light-sensitive film. The energy in the light causes chemical changes in the film of the camera, and chemical changes also occur when light strikes what are called rods and cones on the light-sensitive "film" or retina at the back of the eye. This is, very simply speaking, how light images are received in the eye.

But when it comes to seeing, it helps to think of the eye more in terms of a television camera where the images received are translated into electrical impulses that are transmitted via cable to a screen where a picture is produced instantaneously. In the eye, chemical changes in the rods and cones, caused by the energy in light rays, are translated into electrical impulses which are transmitted along a cable—the optic nerve—to the brain which interprets the impulses and allows you to see a picture, instantaneously, of what you are looking at.

The difference between the eyes and a television camera is that the eye-brain combination is a much more sophisticated system. Eyes have automatic synchronization, focusing, diaphragm control, and interpretation features that are far beyond the capabilities of the best TV equipment. And the eyes have built-in maintenance systems to boot.

The entrance to the eye is covered by a clear, globelike structure called the cornea. The cornea is so clear that it can't be seen easily when you look directly into your eyes, so if you would like to get a good

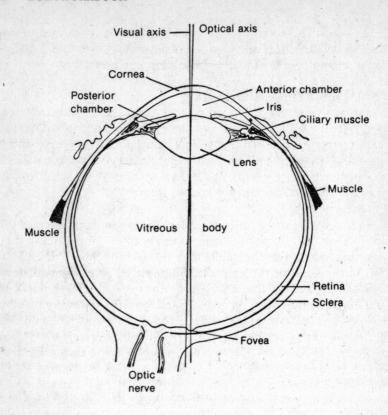

Diagram of the Eye

look at your cornea, stand close to a mirror and shine a small flashlight onto the colored part of your eye from the side. The clear, globe-shaped cornea can easily be seen looking like a spherical cap over the colored part of the eye and the black hole, or pupil, in the center.

The cornea is the first part of the focusing system that light strikes as it enters the eye. Being in the very front of the eye, the corneas are very vulnerable to injuries that can cause severe loss of vision or blindness—a good reason to see that your eyes are well protected when working in potentially dangerous situations.

The amount of light entering the eye is controlled by the iris—the colored part—which is equivalent to the diaphragm in a camera. When there is more light than the eye likes, the iris makes the pupil, or eye opening, smaller. In dim light, the iris draws back, enlarging the pupil to admit as much light as possible. This is an automatic response, or reflex action, and it is one of several reflexes that a doctor looks at when doing a general examination of a patient.

Testing Pupillary Reflex

The pupillary reflex should be strong and rapid. Looking into a mirror, shine the light from a small flashlight into the eye diagonally, from the outside corner. Do not shine the light directly into your eye, and a momentary flash of light will do. As the light strikes your eye you will see the iris instantly contract to make the pupil smaller. When you take the light away, the pupil becomes instantly larger.

Certain diseases and injuries can affect the proper functioning of the irises so that they do not respond to changes in light the way they should. In these cases, the pupils may not change in size when light shines in the eyes, or the pupils may appear to be of unequal sizes. Drugs can also affect the irises' response to light. Heavy doses of opium-derived drugs such as codeine and heroin can cause pinpoint-size pupils and this is one sign that doctors or law-enforcement officers look for when they suspect they are dealing with someone who has recently used these drugs. Other drugs affect the iris in such a way that the pupil openings become quite large. An old drug, belladonna, is one of these and, in fact, got its name from just this phenomenon. *Bella donna* means beautiful woman, and at a time when large pupils and a delicate skin pallor were considered alluring, women probably used the drug to create these conditions. But if they did use belladonna cosmetically, the ladies must have suffered for their beauty, because the drug causes some uncomfortable side effects including blurred vision and an oppressively dry mouth.

As light rays pass the iris they encounter the lens of the eye where they are focused sharply toward the retina at the back of the eye. The eye must adjust in order to focus images on the retina whether the object being looked at is nearby or far away. This happens in a camera when the photographer slightly changes the distance between the lens and the film plane. The photographer's other choice is to change the strength of the lens, and this is done by adding different lenses for objects very near or very far away from the camera.

The eye accommodates itself to seeing objects at different distances by increasing and decreasing the power of its lens. This is accomplished by muscles around the lens which contract to make the lens thicker and its focal length shorter. In a normal eye, light from objects 18 feet or more away will focus on the retina while the muscles around the lens are at rest. Then, when you look at objects closer than 18 feet, the muscles contract to make the lens thicker, which shortens the focus, and an image is formed again exactly on the retina. That is why it is more tiring to do close work than it is to search the horizon for ships at sea. The muscles around the lens must work harder when you do close work.

When the optical system of the eye cannot focus light precisely on the retina for one reason or another, the image formed there is slightly blurred and you need corrective eyeglasses or contact lenses. How well you see is usually spoken of in terms of visual acuity. Visual acuity is the ability to see one object as distinct from another and recognize it. Thus, if you can read the letters on a sign down the street and your friend can't, you have the better visual acuity.

VISUAL ACUITY

No two people see just alike and there is a fairly wide range of what is considered normal vision. But certain arbitrary standards have been set that are a good guide to how well one person can see in relation to another. The familiar chart with letters that get progressively smaller line by line is the most common test used in general screening for visual acuity at distances of more than 18 feet. The chart used most often is called the Snellen scale. Eye-test charts can be obtained inexpensively from most medical supply stores or by writing to the National Society for the Prevention of Blindness, 79 Madison Avenue, New York, NY 10016. There are special E charts and picture charts for preschoolers and those who cannot read. The NSPB charges about 75¢ for adult testing charts while home testing charts for preschool children are free.

Distance Vision.   Eye-test charts are designed to be used at a distance of 20 feet. This gives the first part of the visual acuity rating: 20/20, 20/30, 20/40, and so on. The second or third smallest line of letters from the bottom will be labeled 20/20. If you can read this line of letters easily and accurately, it means that you see as clearly at 20 feet as most people do whose vision is considered normal. If you can read only as far down the chart as the line labeled 20/30, this means that at 20 feet you are only able to see what most people with normal vision can see at 30 feet. If you can read only the line labeled 20/200 when you are standing 20 feet away from the chart, it means your vision is rather severely limited because most people with normal vision can see these letters from 200 feet away.

Going in the opposite direction, if you can read the tiny *20*/15 line, your distance vision is a bit sharper than it is for most people.

Testing Visual Acuity

Place the chart in good light and position yourself 20 feet away from it. (Charts are available to use at 10 feet with a good mirror to produce a reflected image that is 20 feet away.) Be sure there are no shadows and no glare on the chart. Cover one eye gently with a card or your cupped hand. Don't press on the eye you are covering. Read the smallest line of letters you can see clearly. Have someone close to the chart check to see that you are not stumbling over letters or reading them incorrectly. Record the label of the smallest line you can read. Switch eyes and do the same thing. This time read the line backwards to be sure you are not reading from memory. Finally, test with both eyes open.

If you are not experiencing any discomfort when you use your eyes, a test score as low as *20*/40 is generally considered adequately good vision for most purposes, although some occupations require better than *20*/40 vision or vision that can be brought to *20*/20 with correcting lenses. Police and fire departments and the military services are among those that usually require better visual acuity. If you score lower than *20*/40, you should visit an eye doctor for a formal evaluation. If your eyes test in the normal range but one eye tests considerably better than the other, say *20*/20 for one and *20*/40 for the other, you should also get a professional evaluation.

A Rough Test for Distance Vision

A rough but effective way to check the quality of distance vision is simply to compare your ability to read road signs or billboard advertising with someone who is known to have good vision. It can be made a game with children. Predetermine the distance at which a clearly lettered sign is just visible to the person with good vision. Have the person being tested try to read the words with one eye at a time. If there is noticeable difficulty, that is, if the person being tested has to move a good bit closer to the sign than seems necessary, more formal testing should be done.

Blurred distance vision is more often the result of an error in the eye's optical system than a result of a defect in the nerves, blood vessels, or other tissues that serve the eye. The eyeball itself may be a bit too long in relation to the strength of the lens system so that light from distant objects focuses short of the retina. This is what happens in myopia, or nearsightedness. In nearsightedness, as the name implies, distance vision is not as good as it should be and this can be spotted easily with eye-chart testing.

Another error in the optical system, which often goes unnoticed in young people, is hyperopia, or farsightedness. In hyperopia, light tries to focus behind the retina. But this signals the muscles around the lens to shorten the focus, which they do by squeezing the lens to make it a bit thicker. This corrects the error and allows the hyperope to see 20/20 or better, but it keeps the muscles working overtime and can result in fatigue and headaches. With aging, however, a hyperope may begin to experience blurred distance vision because, as one gets older, the accommodation mechanism becomes progressively more inefficient. This blurring will show up—in older people, not in young people—with eye-chart testing.

Near Vision. In addition to testing your vision at 20 feet, you should measure your near point of accommodation. This is the closest point in front of your eyes where you can see an object clearly without blurring or distortion. If you do a good bit of close work—reading, writing, sewing, sorting, assembling, repairing—and if you are approaching forty, it is important for you to understand this near point and to know where it is for you.

Determining Your Near Point of Accommodation
To find your near point, take an ordinary yardstick and rest its end gently against your cheekbone. Hold the yardstick so that it sticks directly out in front of you. Hold some reading material with fairly small print in the other hand. A newspaper, magazine or this book will do. Hold the reading material at a distance along the yardstick where you can read the words easily; then move the page toward you, watching the letters as they become more difficult to read. At some point the words will blur and become difficult to read. Move the page back out until you can read the words comfortably again. Note where this point is on the yardstick. This distance from your eye to the page is your near point of accommodation.

If you are under forty, your near point should be about 12 to 14 inches or closer. In young people the near point can be as close as 3 or 4 inches. If you are past forty and are already wearing a corrective prescription for reading—either reading glasses or bifocals—your near point should also be within the 12- to 14-inch range or shorter when you are wearing your glasses. When the near point moves out beyond

14 inches, as it does inexorably with aging, it becomes inconvenient, uncomfortable, and sometimes dangerous to work without corrective lenses. It is foolhardy to work around fast-moving machinery, for instance, if you are not sure that you can see it clearly at a comfortable working distance. And a day at the office can be sheer misery if you must struggle constantly to find a distance at which you can see your work.

The condition is called presbyopia and it happens to everyone. It is a result of the progressing inefficiency of the accommodation mechanism of the eye mentioned earlier. Reading glasses, or a reading correction added to a prescription you already wear (bifocals), easily solves the problem. If your work requires constant shifting of your eyes from near to intermediate to distant objects, such as a teacher might have to do in shifting from blackboard to students to a book, trifocal lenses that help focus light from three distances are often a practical solution.

In young people the near point is generally not much of a concern, although what happens when a young person does near work is important. We noted that young, farsighted (hyperopic) people can usually see quite well at a distance, but their eye muscles are under constant tension to put images on the retina. The closer the object, the harder the muscles must work. So reading and other near work can put considerably more strain on farsighted eyes than on normal eyes. This will not be noticed as blurred vision; but fatigue, headache, dizziness, and nausea after periods of close work may tip you off that something is amiss. Children with this condition are usually unaware that anything is wrong, but they become understandably reluctant to read or do other near work. Whenever there is undue reluctance to read or do schoolwork, vision should be checked by an eye doctor as a possible cause.

Most people do not have their visual acuity and other functions of seeing checked as often as they should. Children should have their first professional eye examination no later than age three and preferably younger. Certain correctable defects can be corrected only if they are discovered and treated when a child is very young. Eyes should be tested again when a child starts school and then at two-year intervals throughout life. Where adults are concerned, such things as retinal detachments and glaucoma are treated today with extremely high success rates when they are discovered early. When they go undiscovered and untreated they quickly cause irreversible eye damage.

Visual screening for near and distance vision should be a part of the health program in every school. If there is no program in your child's school you may want to contact the National Society for the Prevention of Blindness for information and help in getting one started. With very little training, volunteer nonprofessionals can conduct highly effective visual-screening programs.

Astigmatism.   Astigmatism is another common problem that occurs in the eye's optical system. What happens in astigmatism is that light rays from objects in different planes of vision focus at different points within the eye. That is, when you look at the letter E on the eye chart or on a road sign, for example, you may see the vertical bar of the E more clearly than the cross bars; or, one line of an X may look clearer and darker than the other. This is generally attributed to an error in the shape of the cornea or in the shape of the eyeball itself. Both blurring and distortion can occur with astigmatism and may result in obvious discomfort—headaches, tension, tightness—as the eyes try to cope with focusing different images in different planes.

Testing for Astigmatism

Many cases of astigmatism can be discerned with a simple eye chart you can make yourself. On white paper draw eight pairs of lines that are 45 degrees apart and pointing at a common center, as shown. This results in a sort of circular clock face. Make the lines about 8 inches long and about ¼ inch wide. Use a black felt-tip pen or marking crayon and be sure that all the lines are equally wide and equally black.

Astigmatism Chart

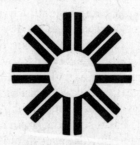

Place the chart in good light about 20 feet away. If you can't see the chart at 20 feet, move closer until you can see the lines. Cover one eye and see if any set of lines looks darker, clearer, or sharper than the set of lines at right angles to it. Repeat with the other eye. If there seems to be a distinct difference in the darkness and clarity of one set of lines over that at right angles to it, then some degree of astigmatism probably exists and a professional evaluation is in order. Most astigmatism can be corrected easily with eyeglasses.

FOR YOUR PERSONAL HEALTH RECORD

1. Check your distance vision. If you wear eyeglasses or contact lenses, check both with and without your correction. Record results and the date. Recheck once a year.

2. Find your near point of accommodation—with and without correcting eyeglasses or contact lenses, if you wear them. Record the results and the date. Recheck once a year. Check every six months if you are approaching forty.

3. Check for astigmatism and record your findings.

4. If you have a professional eye examination, record the findings in detail. Ask your doctor or the optician for a copy of your prescription if you are told eyeglasses are necessary. Keep this as part of your permanent health record.

COORDINATION OF EYE MOVEMENTS

While the optical system of the eye is a genuine wonder by itself, even more wonderful is the rapid communication between the eyes and the brain that enables us to see the world as we do and perform a variety of functions which, if you stop to think about them, should really be impossible. You can look at an object and know if it is near or far away and you can estimate its size at any distance. You can judge textures, from big bumps on the earth called mountains to the little bumps that make the difference between sheer and nubby curtain material.

This happens, in part, because of the brain's ability to change two-dimensional images received by the eyes into three-dimensional visual perception. We say, then, that we have depth perception and the world has form and texture for us because of it. People with only one eye can have an adequate sense of depth and they can judge distances, but it works much better with two eyes—binocular vision, this is called.

Because the eyes are slightly separated, each sees a slightly different image and the brain fuses these into a single, three-dimensional picture. Another feature of binocular vision is the ability of the eyes to move in their sockets in synchronized and coordinated movements in response to either conscious or unconscious commands from the brain. Both these phenomena are easy to observe.

Testing Eye Coordination

Have someone sit holding their head steady, looking straight forward. Ask your subject to follow the motion of your hand as you move it up and down, from side to side, diagonally, and finally, in a circle. The range of motion of the eyes, which is controlled by six paired and opposing muscles in each eye, is quite remarkable. Then, ask your subject to watch your finger as you move it from a distance to the tip of his or her nose. The eyes turn in and down, a movement which is much more obvious in younger people, who can fixate on an object as close as two or three inches from the eyes. Now, hold your finger steady a foot or more away and ask your subject to look at it while moving the head up and down, sideways, and in a circle. Now the eyes remain in one position while the eye sockets and the rest of the head revolve around them. The same muscles are at work.

Observe these eye movements carefully. The eyes should work together smoothly. Especially notice what happens when you move your finger from far to near and back out again. One eye may turn slightly more than the other, or at least the turning may be more noticeable in one eye than the other. But if there are large differences in the movements—one eye turns considerably more than the other, one refuses to turn or follows reluctantly—there may be a muscle imbalance or coordination problem that should be noted and discussed in the course of a professional eye examination.

To prove that your eyes see different images, hold up your finger and with one eye closed align the finger with a distant object. Now switch eyes. The relationship between finger and object shifts noticeably. Open and close your eyes alternately and there is a good bit of jumping around of images.

Generally, one eye is a fixing or dominant eye, while the other obediently turns to fix on the same object the dominant eye is looking at. If this doesn't happen, you may get double vision. Double vision can result from a variety of causes that include too much alcohol, fatigue, muscle imbalance, defects in the eyes' optical system, and perception problems that originate in the brain. Any condition that indicates that the eyes are not working together to see a single image should be reported to the doctor at once.

Determining Your Dominant Eye
Most people have a dominant right eye just as most people have a dominant right hand. And what's more, chances are good that your dominant eye will be on the same side as your dominant hand. To find your dominant or fixing eye, make a circle with your thumb and forefinger—the OK sign. Holding the circle about a foot away from your eyes, and with both eyes open, sight through the circle at some distant object. Close your left eye. If the object is clearly within the circle, you are sighting or fixing with your right eye. If the opposite is true, the object is within the circle with the left eye open and the right shut, you are sighting with your left eye. If you find you can't sight easily with one hand, try using the other.

When the two eyes fail to turn and work together, the condition is known as strabismus. This and other conditions, such as when one eye has much better visual acuity than the other, often cause the brain to suppress vision in one of the eyes. Rather than deal with disparate and confusing images, the brain may prefer to "turn off" one of the pictures. Most people can do this voluntarily when sighting a rifle or when looking through a magnifying glass with one eye only, although both eyes are kept open.

If the brain persistently suppresses the vision in one eye during normal seeing, the suppressed eye will eventually lose its ability to see. This happens more often than it should with young children. Many parents, noticing that a child's eyes are not working together, simply wait for the child to "outgrow" it. This attitude arises from the fact that infants' eyes tend to dissociate, not work together, up to about six months, and then they do outgrow it. But after six months, the eyes should be developed enough to work together, and if they don't the condition should be investigated at once. Vision in a suppressed eye can be lost fairly rapidly, so the sooner it is caught the better. Treatment for this condition is faster and more successful if begun before age three and success rates decline markedly after that. Many ophthalmologists suggest a professional eye examination in infancy and again before age three. And certainly any noticeable crossing or divergence in children's eyes should be investigated at once.

VISUAL FIELD

At the beginning of the chapter we noted that light impulses are picked up and started on their way to the brain by specialized cells called rods and cones that are located on the retina—the light-sensitive "film" at the back of the eye. The retina is about the size of a postage stamp, as thin as onion skin, and loaded with rods and cones, perhaps 150 million or more of them. Rods can only perceive images as black and white while cones can discern color. The most sensitive point on the retina is a small spot near the center called the fovea that is barely 1/50 inch in diameter and packed with cones. It is here that the sharpest vision and most color vision occurs. The eyes stay in constant motion, even when you're not aware of it, in an effort to keep the image of whatever you are looking at focused on this tiny spot.

With one eye closed, stare at the second *n* in the word conce*n*trate. You will see the *e* and the *t* on either side of the *n* rather well, but you will notice that letters beyond that quickly begin to get gray. Your area of sharpest vision and best color discrimination is quite small. But beyond that the total field of vision is surprisingly large, even though you see only in black and white over most of it. You can see almost straight to the side—out of the "corner" of your eye—while looking straight ahead, and you could do as well up and down and to the other side if it weren't for eyebrows, cheekbones, and your nose getting in the way. Since there are diseases of both the eye itself and the brain which tend to reduce the extent of this visual field, it is important that you be familiar with what it is and how far it extends for you. You can do this very simply.

Determining Your Visual Field

Stand a little more than arm's length away from a wall with your right shoulder pointing toward some convenient marker on the wall, a door frame, or the edge of a picture. Choose a small object directly in front of you and some distance away, and stare at it intently. With your left hand, cover your left eye. Now, hold your right hand out from your right side on a level with your eyes. Move your arm just back from the midline and point your fingers forward loosely. Wiggle your fingers and slowly move your arm forward. Continue staring intently at the object in front of you. Resist the temptation to peek at your fingers. After moving your arm just slightly forward of the midline, your wiggling fingers will suddenly come into view even as you are staring straight to the front. This will not be a sharp image, but the motion will be clearly perceived. This is the edge of your visual field on your right side using the right eye.

Stop as soon as you hit this point and look to see where your arm is. It should be about 80 or 85 degrees from a line straight in front of you —about 15 degrees from the midline of your shoulder. Touch the wall. You will be less than 6 inches from your marker. This means you can perceive objects almost directly to the side but not quite. Perform the same test with your wiggling fingers from several angles—above your head, from below, diagonally, and from the nose side. (You will have to change hands when working from the nasal side.) The field from above will only be about 50 degrees and just a little better from the bottom. This is because your eyebrows and cheekbones are in the way. You will manage still less from the side where the nose gets in the way. Test both eyes in the same manner.

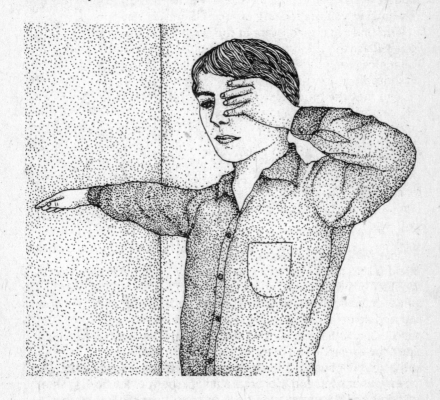

The importance of field of vision is obvious in avoiding danger from the side when driving an automobile, in performing well in sports, and in many occupations that require you to be aware of what's going on at the edges of your visual field. But most important, a contracting field can be a sign of major trouble and must be investigated by an eye doctor as soon as it is suspected.

Tracking Your Visual Field

You can track and keep a record of the outer edges of your visual field if you use a partner to help you. Make a large black spot on a piece of paper—about one inch in diameter—and tape this on a wall at eye level. Try to select a wall that gives you about 6 feet of working room on each side when you stand facing it. Stand about 20 inches away from the wall, cover one eye and stare fixedly at the black dot. The exact distance from the wall doesn't matter, but record it accurately for future reference. If you are much further than 20 inches from the wall, your partner will have to reach further than is comfortable to do the test.

Have your partner place his hand on the wall far enough to the right so that it is outside your field of vision. Then your partner should move his hand in slowly, wiggling the fingers until you can just see the motion. But remember, you are staring at the black spot, not looking sideways for fingers. Call "stop" just as you detect the movement and let your partner mark the place on the wall. Repeat to the left, from above and below and on 45-degree diagonals. Make a sketch on a piece of paper showing the black spot in the center and the distances from it to the places marked on the wall. Label the sketch right eye or left eye as the case may be and keep the data for your personal health record. Be sure you have recorded the distance from your eye to the wall. Do the same thing for the other eye. Test again in about six months, being sure you are the same distance from the wall as before. If there is any marked shrinking of your visual field, you should report the fact to an eye doctor at once.

FOR YOUR PERSONAL HEALTH RECORD

   1. Check the edges of your visual field. Record data obtained and the date.
   2. Recheck once a year and compare with former data. Be sure you have set up the test the same way you did the first time. Report any appreciable loss of field to your eye doctor at once.

Light impulses are carried from the retina of the eye to the brain in a bundle of nerves called the optic nerve. The point at which the optic

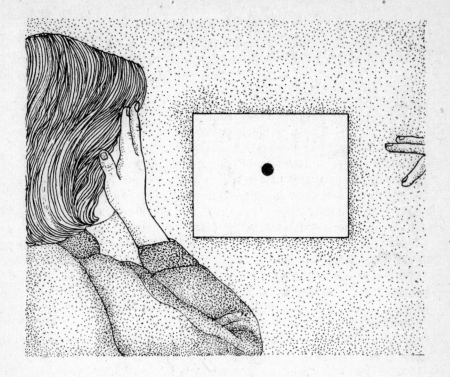

Tracking your Visual Field

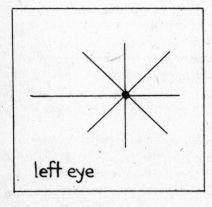

left eye

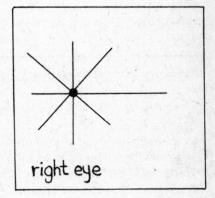

right eye

nerve enters the eyeball is called the optic disc. The disc is like the end of an electric cable with a large number of wires (nerves) being sent out from it to points on the retina where they make contact with the photoreceptor cells (rods and cones). The optic disc itself contains no rods or cones and is, therefore, a blind spot. Everyone has two blind spots, one in each eye. A normal blind spot never gives any trouble in seeing; we're never even aware of it, in fact, but there is an amusing trick that proves it is there.

Blind-spot demonstration

Make a ½-inch-diameter black spot on a piece of stiff paper—a 3 × 5 file card works fine. About 3 inches to the left of the spot make a star, or just an *x* will do. Close your left eye and hold the paper at arm's length with the star directly in front of your right eye. Stare fixedly at the star (or *x*) and bring the paper slowly toward your face. At some point the black spot will disappear. The reason it disappears is that the image of the spot has fallen on the blind spot of your right eye. Move the paper a bit closer and the spot reappears. To find the blind spot of the left eye, stare at the spot with the right eye closed and make the star disappear.

With some patience, a partner to help, and a little practice, you can make use of this phenomenon to map the edge of what is called your central visual field. This is the area in your field of vision affected by your blind spot and it's good to know where it is for the same reason you want to know where your peripheral field ends—a spreading blind spot or the appearance of new blind spots can be an indication of rather serious problems. Here, step by step, is how you can do the mapping.

Mapping Your Blind Spot

1. Make a large black spot (about ½-inch diameter) in the center of a piece of blue-lined notebook paper—the kind you find in an 8½ × 11 looseleaf binder.

2. Make a black star of about the same size on a blank, white, 3 × 5 file card. Putting the star in the middle of one end of the card will be most convenient for the test.

3. Punch a small hole in the center of the star with a sharp pencil point. Gently clean off any ragged edges from around the back of the hole.

4. Arrange a narrow table—18 or 20 inches deep—against a wall. A small typewriter table or a little telephone table is ideal. Find a low chair or stool to sit on. Put a few large books on the table so that when you sit in the chair you can rest your chin comfortably on the books while looking straight ahead at the wall.

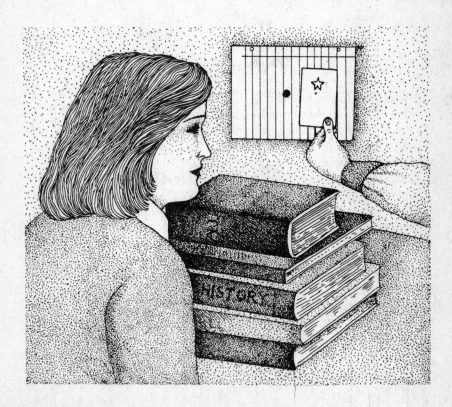

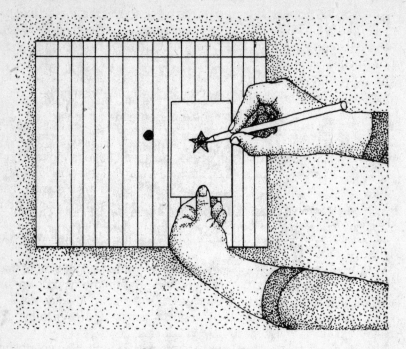

Mapping your Blind Spot

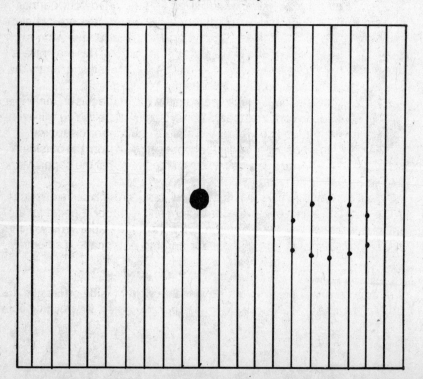

5. Tape the notebook paper with the black spot to the wall so that the spot is directly in front of you at eye level when you are sitting with your chin resting on the books. The blue lines of the notebook paper should run vertically—up and down.

6. Your partner stands beside you holding the card with the star. He should also have a felt-tip pen with a fine point that can make a mark through the hole in the star.

7. Sit in the chair and place your chin on the books. You must maintain this position until the end of the test, so it is a good idea to mark the place where your chin goes in case you have to move. Then you will be able to find the spot again. Find a comfortable position where your eyes are 15 or 20 inches from the wall. Record this distance. The next time you test, your eyes must be at exactly the same distance from the wall.

8. Close your left eye and stare intently at the black spot with your right eye.

9. Choosing a blue line about an inch in from the right side of the paper, your partner should move the black star on the card down this line, slowly, from the top of the paper. At some point the star will disappear. Call "Stop!" and have your partner mark the place by inserting his pen *through* the hole in the star.

10. This is a point where light from the star has fallen on your blind spot. If the star doesn't disappear on the first try, have your partner move a line or two to the left and try again. Be sure you are not succumbing to the temptation to swing your eye toward the moving star. You must stare fixedly at the black spot in front of you. This may take a little practice at first. (If you are not sure what you are looking for, try the blind-spot demonstration described earlier once again.)

11. Work the star down each line from the top of the paper, making a mark each time the star disappears from your visual field. You will eventually arrive at a blue line where the star will no longer disappear.

12. When this happens, begin the process again from the outside of the paper, but work *up* the blue lines from the bottom of the paper. Mark the places where the star disappears as before.

13. When you are finished, the dots will form a rough circle or ellipse to the right and a little below the black spot on the paper. Repeat for the left eye, working the star in from the left side of the paper. You will find that with practice the test goes better and the dots make a smoother pattern.

There may be a dot or two that winds up either inside or outside the general patterns. These can be ignored. If, however, four or five dots fall substantially outside the general pattern, this may be significant and you should bring it to the attention of an eye doctor.

Test again in six months, being sure you position your eyes the same distance from the wall as before. Any changes—additional blind spots or an enlarging pattern—could indicate a developing visual defect and you should be tested professionally at once.

Many conditions, some rare, some rather common, can cause changes in the visual field. Some of these conditions can be treated with an extremely high rate of success if they are caught early enough, which is why it is important for you to be familiar with your normal visual field and thus be aware of any changes as soon as they begin to occur. If you should notice any sudden distortion of visual images, however, or an obvious reduction in any part of the visual field, don't spend a great deal of time making an accurate map of new blind spots. The moment you realize something is wrong, see an eye doctor at once. With modern techniques, defects which only a few years ago would have meant certain blindness are now being treated with routine success. But early treatment is essential. Long delay greatly diminishes chances for good results.

FOR YOUR PERSONAL HEALTH RECORD

  1. Map the edges of your central visual field.
  2. Recheck in six months. Be sure you have set up your test exactly as you did the first time. Report any appreciable change to your eye doctor at once.

RETINAL DETACHMENT AND GLAUCOMA

Of the conditions that can cause a progressive loss of vision, retinal detachment and glaucoma are most worthy of mention here simply because they can be treated so successfully when discovered in time. Retinal detachments can result from disease, injury, or from less obvious and sometimes mysterious causes. The retina separates from the back of the eye with resulting blindness where the detachment occurs. Modern treatment of this disease has been well covered in the press because of its space-age technology involving the use of cryosurgery (freezing) and laser beams. And success rates are as spectacular as the techniques, being as high as 90 percent when the condition is discovered and treatment begun in time. Showers of spots or shadows, or a decreasing field of vision should be investigated at once.

Glaucoma is an insidious eye disease that has been called "the thief of sight." Of two million Americans who have the disease, it is estimated that half are unaware of it, which is a terrible statistic considering that glaucoma can almost always be kept in check easily with eye drops or pills, but if left alone it can cause irreversible blindness.

About four-fifths of the eyeball is filled with a clear jellylike material, the vitreous humor, that exerts just the right amount of pressure to enable the eye to keep its shape. In the very front part of the eye this material is thin and watery and is referred to as the aqueous humour. There is constant circulation of the aqueous humour with new material being secreted as some of it is drained off. If the secretion rate exceeds the drainage rate, then pressure within the eye increases. This is what happens in glaucoma. If the condition is allowed to continue without treatment, the pressure will destroy the delicate retina with resulting blindness. Deterioration of vision is likely to begin around the edge of the visual field, usually starting from the nasal side of the eye. But defects in the field do not necessarily progress in a constant fashion and large cuts in the visual field can occur before the defect is noticed if formal testing is not done on a regular basis. Then, even though the disease is brought under control, the vision which has been lost is gone permanently.

The best test for glaucoma is a direct measurement of the pressure inside the eyeball which is done with an instrument called a tonometer. Tonometer testing should only be done by a doctor or other specially trained person; it is not recommended for home testing. Since glaucoma is much more common in people over the age of forty-five, people approaching the middle years should be tested with a tonometer as a regular part of their annual physical, just as they should be tested with an electrocardiograph to check on the heart. Some doctors recommend that tonometer testing begin as early as thirty-five. If your doctor does not do this test, ask for it. It only takes a minute and is a very minor annoyance to the eye.

The Lions Club International, which has been interested in sight preservation for many years, has begun a program of free tonometer testing in some communities. You might want to contact the Lions Club in your area to find out if it has a program. The National Society for the Prevention of Blindness also sponsors free glaucoma testing in some areas. But find one way or another to have the pressure in your eyes checked regularly. It is important.

CATARACT

Cataract is a disease that affects the eyes of many older people. There are some conditions that cause cataracts in young people—such as congenital cataracts in infants that may result from a mother having had German measles during pregnancy—but the majority of cataracts occur in people over sixty. A cataract is a clouding of the lens of the eye which generally develops over a period of years, although some are known to develop in a matter of months. It begins as a very mild turbidity in the lens, perhaps in just a spot or two, and then as time goes on the lens admits less and less light into the eye. This will result in hazy vision which is likely to show up in eye-chart testing, or it will simply become apparent that sight is not as sharp as it used to be. Night driving may become increasingly difficult because light from approaching cars is diffused by the cloudiness in the lens, producing a dazzling effect.

The exact mechanism that results in cataract is unknown and the treatment consists of surgically removing the cloudy lens. It is an operation that is performed routinely with little risk and only a brief hospital stay. Then, with the help of glasses, contact lenses, or a plastic lens implant, vision is dramatically restored.

SOME OTHER IMPORTANT OBSERVATIONS

There are some vision problems which have nothing to do with the eye itself. The eye may be perfectly intact and theoretically functional, yet blind because of a defect in the brain. This is called cortical blindness since the cause originates in the cortex of the brain. Tumors of the pituitary gland may also impinge on vision connectors causing defects in the visual field. Problems of perception also originate in the brain; that is, the brain, for reasons that remain a mystery, does not process some of the information it receives from the eye in a way that corresponds to the way most other people see things. This happens frequently enough in children who are learning to read and write to cause considerable concern among educators. In one condition, known as dyslexia, letters are seen reversed or upside down. Sometimes it is a temporary confusion that a child outgrows very quickly, but other times it persists into adulthood.

Testing for Dyslexia

You can test for indications of dyslexia by asking a child to read some fairly simple material to you. Observe the kinds of mistakes the child makes. The dyslexic will tend to confuse the lower case letters *d* and *b* or the letters *p* and *b*. Some dyslexics will pronounce the sounds of individual letters easily and then become inextricably confused when they are put together in even simple words. Check the child's writing, too, for reversals and inversions.

Some educators have ventured a guess that as much as **25** percent of the school population may experience some degree of perception difficulty and they suggest that more teachers should be aware of the problem. This does not mean that these children lack intelligence. On the contrary, children with perception problems are frequently somewhat brighter than average but have trouble expressing their intelligence because of the perception problem. Special teaching programs have been developed to help dyslexics to read efficiently, so if you suspect this condition in your child, have it investigated professionally, bring it to the attention of the school principal, and then be sure something is done about it.

Following are other observations that should be made of children's seeing habits. If a child does not seem to be seeing efficiently, it should be looked into by an eye doctor at once.

- Does the child frown excessively?
- Does the child squint when looking at distant objects even when not in bright sunshine?
- Does the child blink excessively, manipulate the eyebrows, or grimace a lot when doing close work?
- Does the child make motions in front of the eyes as if trying to brush away something?
- Does the child complain that letters move or run together?
- Does the child often fail to see what others see?
- Do teachers complain about inattention during reading or blackboard activities, or complain that Johnny is a bright boy but doesn't do as well as he should?

In addition to watching children's eyes, everyone should become familiar with their own eyes, how they see and what normal eyes look like. Any unusual condition that persists for more than a day or so should be called to the attention of a doctor. Some unusual conditions not mentioned before:

- Unusual sensitivity to light
- Persistent pain, burning or itching
- Headaches associated with using the eyes

• Redness of the eyeball; marks or bumps
• Anything unusual about the eyelids, inside or outside
• Excessive tearing or unusual discharges; eyelids that stick together
• Change in pupil size; unequal pupil sizes; very large or very small
  pupils

The visual acuity test, using the letter chart, is the most useful tool for a quick general-vision evaluation. If your vision is poorer than the 20/20 to 20/40 range, you should consult an eye doctor. The other tests we have described are extremely useful in keeping track of your eyes over the years and between the times that you see your doctor. But if you develop any untoward symptoms such as blurring, distortion, haloes around lights, tunnel vision, or other restrictions and cuts in the visual field, do not try to diagnose the defect yourself. Consult an eye doctor. In the case of glaucoma, retinal detachments, and certain other conditions, delay in consulting a doctor can result in irretrievable vision loss that could have been prevented.

CHAPTER 3

TESTING THE NERVOUS SYSTEM

The nervous system, consisting of the brain, the spinal cord, and nerves which stream out to every part of the body is unquestionably the most awesome structure of the human body. The central nervous system functions as the body's command headquarters, processing incoming information, controlling body functions, and making decisions at a rate that would blow a fuse on the most sophisticated computer.

Yet despite its staggering complexity, a basic evaluation of the nervous system is carried out using very simple equipment. Some tests are done by observation alone. Some require a simple hat pin, some a flashlight, and some a little rubber hammer. Unlike other medical specialists, neurologists rely less on X rays, complicated tests, and elaborate equipment than on close observation and careful reasoning. The blink of an eye—or the absence of a blink—is worth a thousand X rays to the neurologist. The simplest reflex response tells a skilled specialist volumes about the subject's nerve pathways.

Obviously, it takes years of training and experience to detect subtle symptoms of neurologic disorders and interpret their significance. Still, it is possible to perform a fairly comprehensive evaluation of the nervous system through self-testing. The simple tests and observations described later on in this chapter should help you spot potentially troublesome abnormalities that should be brought to the attention of a specialist, and will also tell you when things are normal and working well. First, however, a brief review of the anatomy of the nervous system will give you a better understanding of the tests which follow.

THE NERVOUS SYSTEM

The Brain.   Of all the organs in the body, the brain is the last to give up its secrets. Like outer space, the brain is one of the "last frontiers" left to penetrate. Many aspects of brain function are not at all understood, and there is a growing body of evidence that the brain is more than a super-complicated computer made up of nerve cells and connecting elements. Recent findings suggest that the brain probably also secretes a number of subtle, hormone-like substances which tell the master endocrine gland—the pituitary—what to do.

Microscopically, the brain consists of about 30 billion neurons, or nerve cells, supported by a fine network of glial cells, plus a wealth of blood vessels to provide nourishment for the cells.

There are two great lobes of the brain, called the cerebral hemispheres, which lie adjacent to each other and fill most of the skull. Deep inside these cerebral hemispheres is an open space filled with a watery substance called cerebral spinal fluid. This fluid fills the hollow

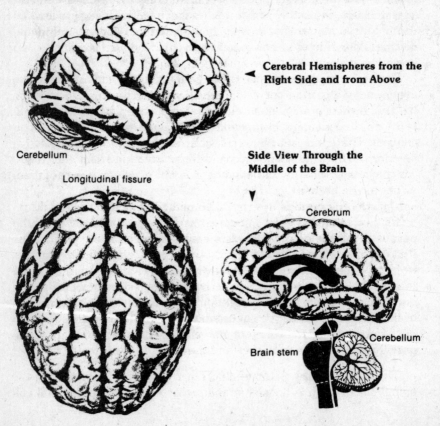

◄ **Cerebral Hemispheres from the Right Side and from Above**

Cerebellum

Longitudinal fissure

Side View Through the Middle of the Brain

▼

Cerebrum

Cerebellum

Brain stem

spaces in the brain called the ventricles and also the space surrounding the spinal cord. If a doctor does a procedure called a spinal tap, he is taking a small sample of this fluid for analysis.

The cerebral hemispheres control virtually all the higher functions including reason, speech, memory, smell, taste, vision, and movement. One hemisphere is always dominant over the other. If you are right-handed, your left hemisphere is probably dominant; if you are left-handed, your right hemisphere is likely the dominant one. The dominant hemisphere usually controls speech. This and other general areas of the brain which control certain functions have been well established. For example, the sense of smell is located up near the front of the cerebral hemispheres, and the sense of vision near the back. Muscle control is located along the sides.

The next major segment of the brain, called the cerebellum, sits beneath and toward the rear half of the great cerebral hemispheres and is also divided into two sections. The cerebellum controls functions of which you are generally unaware, such as balance and kinesthesia. Kinesthesia is the ability to know where a part of your body is located without looking at it. That is to say, you know that your arm is hanging down at your side or pointing up in the air without looking at it. You know this because you have kinesthetic sense.

The final part of the brain is the brain stem. This is actually the upper end of the spinal cord and is shaped like the rounded knob on the end of a straight-handled cane. The brain stem goes up just in front of the cerebellum and tucks up underneath and into the cerebral hemispheres. The brain stem controls what are referred to as vegetative functions. These include, among others, breathing and heartbeat, which continue whether or not you are awake or asleep, aware of them or not aware of them.

If part of the brain is destroyed, some body function usually disappears. For example, when someone has a stroke, the blood supply to part of one of the cerebral hemispheres is usually cut off. This means that the part of the brain nourished by this particular blood vessel dies from lack of oxygen. It does this in very short order—usually no more than five minutes without oxygen is enough to destroy brain cells. And once they are gone, they are gone for good. There is no regrowth. The brain may learn to adapt or get along without certain cells by setting up compensating networks of nerve connections, but there is no growth of new brain cells after an injury.

The Spinal Cord.   Continuing down from the brain stem is the spinal cord, which is housed in and protected by the bony spinal column. The spinal cord is sometimes thought of as simply a cable, or trunkline, of nerve fibers connecting the brain with the rest of the body, but it is actually much more than this. The spinal cord carries out some functions which might ordinarily be thought of as brain functions. For example, the simple reflex arc is actually a spinal-cord function. If you tap someone's knee in the right place, the leg jerks. It's not the brain telling the leg to jerk, however, but the spinal cord. This simple knee-jerk reaction is called an arc because the nerves which receive the tap from the hammer send the signal to the spinal cord; the signal is processed right there, and the message directing the muscle to jerk is sent right back. You don't need your brain to jerk your knee when it is tapped.

The Peripheral Nerves.   The final element of the nervous system, after the brain and the spinal cord, consists of the peripheral nerves which run uninterrupted from connections in the spinal cord to all parts of your body. Thirty-one pairs of nerve bundles branch out from the spinal cord. Almost half are sensory nerves which convey information *to* the brain; the rest are motor nerves which transmit orders *from* the brain to the muscles. These are the final functioning messengers in the nervous system. More than any other part of the nervous system, the peripheral nerves can be thought of as a network of wires which connect the various organs and extremities of the body with the brain.

There is never just a single nerve connecting the spinal cord to a limb, however; there are many, many of them. Each small, special part of the muscle has its own nerve. What anatomists and surgeons often refer to as a single nerve, such as the large radial nerve in the arm, is not a single nerve at all but a bundle of nerves. If the entire bundle is interrupted, those fingers which it controls will hang limply and not work at all. If the bundle is only cut partway through, some functions of some of the fingers will probably remain. It all depends on which of the nerves inside the bundle are interrupted.

EXAMINING YOUR NERVOUS SYSTEM

The Cranial Nerves.   When a neurologist examines your nervous system, he usually begins with a special set of nerves called the cranial nerves. These are special nerves because, instead of coming off the spinal cord as all other major nerves do, the cranial nerves emanate directly from the base of the brain. There are twelve pairs of cranial nerves, with one nerve of each pair for the right side of the body and one for the left.

Because nerves branching off some cranial nerves serve different organs, a single cranial nerve may control several body functions. Testing for one function does not mean that the total nerve bundle is in good working order. And since muscles and nerves are so closely related in their functioning, it is often difficult to know when a dysfunction is the fault of a muscle or a nerve. So while the following tests are interesting and informative, it should be kept in mind that they are not of themselves conclusive. Whenever some lack of function or abnormal functioning of a body part or organ is noticed it should, of course, be called to a doctor's attention.

The first cranial nerve is the olfactory nerve, which controls smell.

Testing the Olfactory Nerve

Some neurologists carry little bottles of peppermint and other scents, and ask the patient to distinguish between two scents, such as peppermint and almond. You can easily perform this same test yourself with food flavorings. Vanilla, peppermint, almond, and cherry extracts can be found in the spice section of any supermarket. Place each bottle in a small bag, twisting the top of the bag so that only the mouth of the bottle is exposed. Smell each of them. If you can correctly identify all four scents, your first cranial nerve is said to be intact.

The second cranial nerve is the optic nerve. This is the nerve bundle which leads out from the back of each eyeball, crosses its partner a little way behind the eyes and under the brain, and makes its way toward the rear part of the brain. The vision and visual field tests described in the chapter on vision testing are actually tests of the second cranial nerve. If you have good vision (with glasses, if necessary) and full visual fields, you can say that your second cranial nerve is intact.

The third, fourth, and sixth cranial nerves control the muscles that govern eye movement. These three nerves—the oculomotor (III), the trochlear (IV), and the abducens nerve (VI)—work together to move the eyes in a coordinated fashion.

Testing the Nerves Which Control Eye Movement

A simple test of the third, fourth, and sixth cranial nerves is to have the subject stare intently at a small object, such as the tip of a pencil. Moving the object from side to side and up and down, observe how the subject follows it with the eyes. The head itself should not move at any time during this test—only the eyes.

If the eyes move fully and in coordination with each other from side to side and up and down, and double vision does not occur during any of these motions, you can be quite certain that the third, fourth, and sixth cranial nerves are functioning correctly.

If double vision should suddenly occur during this test, it may indicate some degree of malfunction of one of the muscles which move the eyes. Since these three nerves work together, it is often difficult to determine exactly which of the nerves is at fault, or if it is a muscle weakness, without sophisticated testing by an ophthalmologist. For example, an inability to move the eye outward only, suggests a problem with the sixth nerve. Similarly, a drooping of one eyelid may be due to an interruption of the third (oculomotor) nerve near its ending in the brain.

Testing for Malfunction of the Third Cranial Nerve

If movement in one eyeball is sluggish or nonexistent and the pupil does not react to light, this may indicate problems with the third cranial nerve.

To test for this function, shine a flashlight into one eye, and then the other, for a second or two each time. The pupils of *both* eyes should constrict in response to light shined into either eye.

With problems of the third nerve, the pupil often remains fully dilated and unresponsive to light, although this is not the only reason that the pupil may not react to light. For a more detailed discussion of the pupillary reflex, refer to the chapter on vision testing.

The fifth cranial nerve, called the trigeminal because it has three branches, controls (among other things) the sensation of light touch over the face and much of the scalp.

Testing for Light Touch Sensation

You can test for fifth-nerve function using a wisp of cotton. You will need an assistant to help you. With the subject's eyes closed, the examiner takes a wisp of cotton and lightly touches it to the subject's face at different points. The subject reports when a sensation is felt. An inability to sense two or more touches is an abnormal finding.

Sensation over the white part of the eye is also a fifth-nerve function that you can test. Like the skin of the face and scalp, the eye surface is extremely sensitive to touch when the fifth cranial nerve is intact.

Testing the Scleral Reflex

To test the scleral reflex, ask your partner to take a twisted wisp of cotton and touch it to the white part of the eye. You should immediately blink. When you do this test, choose an object to look at and stare at it intently. When you are staring at this object, your partner should bring the wisp of cotton in toward the eye from the very outer edge, so that you do not see it coming. If you blink when the cotton is touched to the eye and you are quite certain that you did not see the cotton coming, then your fifth cranial nerve is normal.

If the fifth nerve is impaired, the subject will not feel the cotton against the eye that is touched and the blink response will not occur in *either* eye. If, on the other hand, the eyelid of the *other* eye closes when the cotton touches the white part of one eye, this indicates a lesion, or impairment, of the seventh cranial nerve which controls the eyelid. In such cases the subject will attempt to blink *both* eyes in response to the sensation of touch on the eye. But because of the impaired seventh nerve, the lid on the affected side does not work.

The seventh cranial nerve is the facial nerve and, among other functions, it controls the muscles of expression. When you smile or frown, you are using your seventh cranial nerve.

Detecting Disorders of the Facial Nerve
One of the earliest signs of a seventh-nerve disorder is a flattening of the muscles of one side of the face. This is due to a loss of muscle tone resulting from a decrease in the nerve impulses coming through the damaged seventh nerve. (Each nerve, you will recall, is actually a *pair* of nerves, with each half of the pair supplying one side of the body. Unless both nerves in the pair are damaged, impairment of one nerve affects only one side of the body.) A crooked smile, in which one side of the mouth crinkles naturally while the other side remains relatively expressionless, is a telltale sign of a facial-nerve disorder.

Another early indication of seventh-nerve disorder is an eye that appears to be slightly wider open than the other eye. In more advanced cases, it becomes difficult to close the affected eye at all.

The seventh nerve also controls the taste sensation in the front two-thirds of the tongue. Just as every shade in the rainbow is based on some combination of the three primary colors—red, yellow, and blue—so too are the countless tastes which we enjoy composed of a mingling of four primary tastes—salt, sour, sweet, and bitter. Thus you can check this aspect of seventh-nerve function by distinguishing among these four primary tastes.

Testing Taste Sensation

In little cups, prepare separate solutions of each of the four primary taste sensations: a strong solution of ordinary sugar in water, a strong solution of ordinary table salt in water, a concentrated solution of instant coffee,* and either lemon juice or vinegar. Rinse your mouth with water before beginning the test and between testing each of the four primary tastes:

Take a cotton-tipped swab, dip it in one of the solutions, and touch it to one side of your tongue fairly far forward but not at the very tip. (Note: When doing this test, it is important to place a very small amount of the fluid well to one side of the midline of the tongue. If a trace of fluid seeps across to the other side, you will not have a reliable test because you may actually be tasting the solution with the other side of your tongue.) Test each of the four taste sensations on one side of the tongue, and then repeat and test on the other side. You should be able to taste each solution correctly and separately on each side of your tongue. If you cannot distinguish between any two of them, you may have a problem with the seventh nerve.

The eighth cranial nerve is the auditory nerve, and it has two functions. One function is hearing: If your hearing is adequate as defined by the tests in the "Ear, Nose, Mouth, Throat, and Neck" chapter, then that aspect of eighth-nerve function is normal. Part of the eighth nerve also leads to the semicircular canals in the inner ear, which affect balance and position sense. While balance and position sense are also assisted by feedback from the muscle system, you can get a pretty accurate assessment of this aspect of eighth-nerve function with the following simple test.

Testing Balance and Position Sense

Stand with your feet together, your eyes closed and your arms down at your sides. Direct your partner to give you a sudden, gentle push backward, forward, or to one side. If you have a normal balance mechanism, your partner will not have to catch you to prevent you from falling; instead, you will immediately correct for the unexpected shove. Disorders of this function of the eighth nerve are usually associated with feelings of dizziness and some degree of hearing loss.

Disorders of the ninth, tenth, eleventh, and twelfth cranial nerves

---

*One teaspoon of instant coffee with two tablespoons of hot water.

are harder to pinpoint because their individual functions are difficult to isolate. For instance, the ninth cranial nerve controls a number of functions that are shared by the tenth and eleventh nerves. Similarly, disorders affecting the ninth and tenth cranial nerves may also affect the eleventh and twelfth, and vice versa. Isolated lesions, or impairments, of these four nerves are quite unusual. Within this network of shared functions, however, there are also some functions which are controlled individually by the last four cranial nerves. These lend themselves nicely to home testing, and provide a basic assessment of each of these nerves.

The ninth cranial nerve regulates two functions of its own—one is taste on the back third of the tongue, and the other is sensation in the back of the throat.

To check taste sensation on the back third of the tongue, use the same four solutions you prepared to test seventh-nerve function (taste on the front two-thirds of the tongue). Follow the same procedure described above, only this time place the drops of solution on the rear third of your tongue. Be sure you test far enough back. You will need a partner to help you. Again, test both sides of the tongue, being careful not to test too close to the midline. You should be able to taste each solution separately and correctly on each side of the rear third of your tongue. If you cannot distinguish between any two of them, you may have a problem with the ninth nerve.

Testing Sensation in the Throat

To test for sensation on the back wall of the pharynx, or throat, you will need a thin straw with a bit of cotton attached to one end. Open your mouth wide and have your partner *gently* rub the wisp of cotton against the back of your throat. To get your tongue out of the way, say "aah." Be sure your partner does not poke too hard; a light touch is all that is needed to determine if there is sensation in this area. Some people have a very active gag reflex and will be made extremely uncomfortable by the lightest touch. Others will be able to tolerate some stroking. Both responses are normal. An absence of response, however, is not normal and may indicate ninth-nerve malfunction.

Stroking the back of the throat normally produces gagging. The presence of a gag reflex is one indication that the tenth cranial nerve, called the vagus, is also functioning. The vagus nerve participates in a great many internal functions. Parts of the vagus extend all the way down to the stomach, and are involved in the secretion of stomach acid. Other branches of this nerve control some of the muscles in the palate which help form normal speech sounds. If, over a period of weeks or months, your speech develops a slightly nasal quality which you are unable to control, this may be a sign of a problem with the vagus nerve. If indeed this is happening, the uvula should deviate to one side. The uvula is the little tongue of tissue which hangs down from the back of the palate, or roof, of the mouth. If there is a nasal quality to the speech, and the uvula deviates to one side, this is suggestive of a vagus-nerve disorder.

The eleventh cranial nerve, referred to as the spinal accessory nerve, controls certain muscles in the shoulders. You can easily check this aspect of eleventh-nerve function by asking your partner to help you perform the following test.

Testing the Spinal Accessory Nerve

To test the eleventh cranial nerve, raise both your shoulders as if shrugging them, but instead of lowering them, hold them elevated. Now have your partner push down hard on both shoulders at the same time, exerting an equal amount of force on both sides. If one shoulder can be pushed down with relative ease while the other still offers good resistance, there may be some impairment of the eleventh cranial nerve.

The twelfth and final cranial nerve is the hypoglossal nerve, which controls tongue movement.

Testing the Hypoglossal Nerve

To test the twelfth cranial nerve, look into a mirror and stick your tongue out. Normally, your tongue protrudes straight out, though a slight deviation to one side is not uncommon. If, however, your tongue protrudes crookedly to one side of the mouth or the other, this suggests a lesion of one side of the twelfth cranial nerve. When *both* sides of this nerve are affected, it is difficult to stick out the tongue at all. In either case, you would probably notice a clumsiness of the tongue which would show up in your speech.

THE SPINAL NERVES

In addition to the twelve pairs of cranial nerves which stem directly from the base of the brain, there are thirty-one pairs of nerves which branch off from the spinal cord to various parts of the body. Unlike the cranial nerves which we evaluated one by one, these spinal nerves, as they are called, are intially tested as a system according to three broad

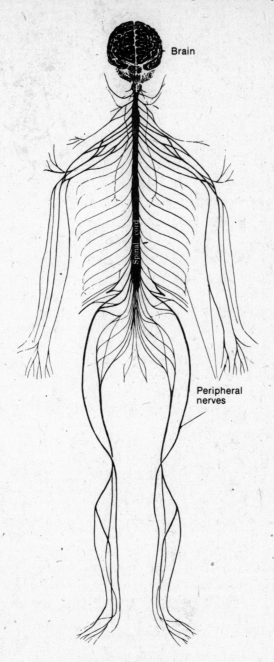

Brain

Spinal cord

Peripheral
nerves

The Spinal Nerves

areas of function: (1) sensory functioning, (2) motor functioning, and (3) mental functioning. You can make a good general assessment of your own nervous system by performing the following tests which check these three functions. Defects revealed by any of these tests should be brought to the attention of a neurologist for more in-depth examination.

Sensory Functioning.   Sensory input provides the nervous system with a wealth of information that enables us to distinguish between sandpaper and silk or hot and cold, to "see" the shape of an object by touch alone, and to know where our hands and feet are and what they are up to even when we can't see them. This kind of information comprises our most basic link with the world around us.

The sensation of touch is easily tested with a simple hatpin, a wisp inputs to the nervous system. Simply stated, it works like this: Special sensing or sensory cells near the surface of the skin detect sensations of touch such as hot or cold, firm pressure or light pressure, smoothness or roughness, and so on, and transmit this information to the brain or spinal cord. The brain or spinal cord then sends back messages through special motor cells instructing the body how to respond—by pulling one's hand away from a flame, for example.

The sensation of touch is easily tested with a simple hat pin, a wisp of cotton, and so on as described further on. Interpreting these tests, however, is not a cut-and-dried matter. There is a wide variation of normal response to sensory inputs from one person to another. The touch of a magician, a surgeon, a pianist, a safecracker, a pickpocket, or a card sharp is likely to be more acute than that of the average person, yet all are within the normal range of response. Bear in mind, too, that some parts of your body are more discriminating than others. For instance, the fingertips are more sensitive than the back, the lips more than the top of the head, and the elbows more than the shin. Thus you would be mistaken to conclude that your sensory system was impaired simply because your lips detected a lighter touch than your shin. If, on the other hand, you discover that one foot is considerably more sensitive to touch than the other, this may be a significant finding. Many nervous-system disorders affect one side of the body more than the other; thus a marked difference in sensory response from side to side should be viewed with suspicion.

Superficial or light touch is very different from the firm pressure of, say, a handshake. Testing this sensation requires an assistant with a delicate touch; even light pressure exerted by a finger or hand in administering the test should be avoided.

Testing Tactile Sensation

Using a wisp of cotton or a soft, camel's hair brush, have your assistant lightly touch or brush various areas of your arms and legs, first on one side, and then the corresponding points on the other side of the body. With your eyes closed, report each time a light touch sensation is felt. In rating your response, try to compare your sensitivity from side to side. A consistent pattern of missed responses on one side of the body is more significant than random misses on both sides.

Superficial pain sensation is another distinct sensory input to the nervous system. Superficial pain is merely a light, fleeting irritation of the surface of the skin, and not a deep or throbbing pain such as you would experience with a cut or a minor burn.

Testing Superficial Pain Sensation

A light pinprick is usually used to check superficial pain sensation. You will need a large hatpin with a little knob at one end for this test, and an assistant.

With your eyes closed, ask your assistant to lightly touch various places on your arms and legs, sometimes with the point of the hatpin and sometimes with the blunt, knobby end. Pay particular attention to examining hands and feet. Report each time you feel a touch, specifying whether it feels sharp or dull.

You should be correct most of the time. Your assistant should retest any areas where you give an incorrect report. Areas in which you consistently give an incorrect report, or fail to perceive any sensation at all, should be brought to the attention of your doctor.

Two-point discrimination is a slight variation of the superficial pain test. The objective here is to ascertain how far apart two simultaneous pinpricks must be separated before you are aware of being touched in two places rather than one.

Testing Two-point Discrimination

This test requires a drawing compass with an interchangeable point/pencil on each leg. Instead of a point on one leg and a pencil lead on the other, as you would use to draw a circle or an arc, you want a fairly sharp point on each leg of the instrument.

Beginning with the two compass points ½ inch apart, instruct your assistant to lightly touch various areas of your body, sometimes with one point and sometimes with both points. When touching both points of the compass to the skin, the examiner should take care that the two points touch the skin at precisely the same instant. With the compass legs ½ inch apart, you will probably find it difficult if not impossible to tell when you are being touched in one place or in two. As the examiner widens the distance between the two points, however, you should be able to report when your skin is touched with two points instead of one. You will find that the distance required for two-point discrimination varies considerably over different parts of the body. On the back, for example, the points have to be at least 2½ inches apart before most people can detect two distinct touches.

Two-point discrimination also varies from one person to another. Thus, in evaluating your results, you should again compare your responses from one side of the body to the other. If you score consistently better on the left side than on the right side, or vice versa, this would be considered an abnormal finding and should be brought to the attention of your doctor.

Testing another sensory input to the nervous system, called stereognostic sense, checks your ability to "decode" sensory information. Stereognostic sense allows you to identify an object by touch alone, without looking at it.

Testing Stereognostic Sense

You can test this sense by providing your assistant with an assortment of small objects such as a penny, a quarter, a fifty-cent piece, a key, a marble, a safety pin, and a ring. Ask your assistant to place these objects in your hand one at a time. With your eyes closed, you should be able to report which object you are holding without looking at it. If you can do this, then you have normal stereognostic sense. You should also have normal two-point discrimination since these two functions really go together.

The ability to detect hot and cold sensations and react appropriately is one of the nervous system's most important sensory inputs. Without it, our body could be irreparably damaged before the smell of singed flesh or the tingling numbness of frostbite alerted our brain to take action. It is no coincidence that one of the earliest words in every baby's vocabulary is "hot!"

Our skin registers different temperature sensations through special nerve endings, some of which respond to cold and falling temperatures, and others to heat and increasing warmth. The heaviest concentration of cold receptors lies in exposed areas like the face, with emphasis on the tip of the nose, the eyelids, lips, and forehead. Parts of the chest, abdomen, and genitals are also highly sensitive to cold. That's why it's always easier to get your feet wet than the rest of your body when you go swimming. You are more sensitive to warmth, on the other hand, on the hairy parts of your head, around your kneecaps, and on your tongue.

You can check to determine that both hot and cold nerve receptors are in good working order with a simple test, as follows.

Testing Temperature Sensation

Temperature sensation can be tested using two test tubes or two of the tubes used to package expensive cigars. Fill one tube with cold water and the other with hot water, about as hot as it comes out of the tap. Have your assistant lightly touch these tubes to various parts of your body, sometimes one tube and sometimes the other.

You should be able to report with your eyes closed whether the hot or the cold tube is touching you. In some neurological disorders, a person may lose the sensation of cold altogether, but still be able to sense warmth. In such cases, ice cubes placed on the skin will feel warm.

Position sense is the ability to know where various parts of your body are without looking. This is possible because impulses from special nerve cells, called sensing or sensory cells, feed signals into the central nervous system that let you know almost instantly that you've raised your hand or moved your foot. You can check position sense in both your arms and legs in the following manner.

Testing Position Sense

Close your eyes and touch the tip of your nose with your index finger, first with one hand and then with the other. Start with your arm extended straight out and bring it slowly in toward the nose. A near miss counts as passing, particularly if you can improve your performance with just a little practice.

Position sense in the legs is usually tested by the heel-to-shin test. While sitting in a chair with your eyes closed, touch the heel of one foot to the shin of the opposite leg and run it up and down a bit. If you can do this accurately with each foot, position sense in the legs is normal. As with the finger-to-nose test, your performance may improve slightly with a little practice.

A final test you can perform to check sensory functioning of the nervous system has to do with movement sense. To test this, you will again need your assistant.

Testing Movement Sense

Ask your assistant to passively move one of your fingers or toes while you have your eyes closed. Your assistant moves one of your fingers or toes up or down or to one side or the other just a little, being very careful not to touch one of the adjacent digits during the examination. Each time a movement is made, you report the direction of the movement. You should be able to distinguish a movement of less than a quarter of an inch in any direction without too much trouble.

Motor Functioning.   The nervous system controls motor functioning—that is, body movement—by signaling the muscles to relax or contract. It does this by sending impulses from the brain or spinal cord to the muscles through special nerve cells called motor cells. The fine fibers that trail out from each motor cell branch off at their endpoints to make contact with fine strands of muscle. The impulses seen through these motor fibers trigger the release of tiny amounts of a chemical which starts the muscle contracting. When the impulses cease coming, the muscle relaxes. Motor function, then, or body movement, is initiated by these special motor nerves which direct muscle action.

Any abnormality of the motor system could, of course, be due to a problem with the muscles themselves, and testing of this aspect of motor activity is covered in the chapter dealing with bones, muscles, and joints. A neurologist, however, will perform special tests to determine that the nervous system is doing its job in directing motor activity. Some of these tests you can do yourself.

The most familiar of all neurologic tests, the knee-jerk reflex, tests the nerves supplying the knee, or patellar, tendon. As noted earlier in this chapter, the knee-jerk test is actually a test of a nerve loop to the spinal cord. The knee-jerk reaction is called a simple reflex arc because the nerves which receive the tap from the little rubber hammer send the signal to the spinal cord; the signal is processed right there and the message directing the muscle to jerk is sent right back. The absence of the knee-jerk reflex is usually a sign of nerve damage, particularly if it is missing on one side only.

Reflex testing is usually done using a small, rubber-headed hammer. In the United States, the head of this hammer is usually triangular in shape and either the wide or the pointed end is used, depending upon the preference of the examiner. There is, however, wide variation in the shape of these hammers. In practice, almost any little weight on the end of a short arm will do. If you wish to purchase a reflex hammer, they are widely available at medical supply stores and are relatively inexpensive. If you are careful and gentle, any small tack hammer will do. Do not use a large carpenter's hammer or other dangerous tool. With practice, some people can learn to use the side of their open hand as a kind of hammer.

Testing the Knee-jerk Reflex

The knee-jerk test is best carried out with some help from an assistant.

1. Sit on a table so that your legs swing freely from the knee joint, with your knees bared.

2. Locate your kneecap with your fingers. You will easily be able to identify this more or less round bone which sits right over the knee.

3. Next, locate a bony prominence an inch or so below the kneecap. This is the top end of the large bone in your lower leg. In the very front part of your leg you will feel a fairly stiff cord running in the short space between the bottom of the kneecap and the top of the leg bone. You should actually be able to put your thumb and index finger on either side of this cord. You are now holding the tendon you are about to test. Mark this point with an X using a felt-tip pen.

4. With your legs totally relaxed, ask your assistant to briskly tap each knee at the point you have marked. It is very important to relax or the test will not work properly. Remember, it is a *tap* you deliver, not a blow.

5. In most people, if the test is done correctly, the lower leg will immediately give a little jerk.

The normal response in this test is extremely variable. Some people have very active knee jerks and others have such inactive knee jerks that it is difficult to elicit any response at all from the test. If you are having difficulty obtaining a knee-jerk reaction, it sometimes helps to hook your hands together, hold them up in front of your chest, and then try as hard as you can to pull them apart. While you are pulling as hard as you can, your assistant should repeat the test. This increase in general muscle tone often strengthens the knee-jerk response in those who normally have a relatively weak response. The most important observation, however, is not the strength of the response, but rather equality of response on the two sides. Both sides should be about the same. A knee-jerk response which is substantially more active on one side than on the other is abnormal and a doctor's opinion should be sought.

Other tendon reflexes can be tested in much the same way. The Achilles' tendon, for instance, responds well to a simple ankle-jerk reflex test. Like the knee jerk, this is best carried out with some help from an assistant.

Testing the Ankle-jerk Reflex

1. Sit on the edge of a table so that your legs swing freely from the knee joint, with your feet and lower legs bared.

2. Locate the Achilles' tendon with your fingers: first identify the heel bone on your foot. Just above the heel bone, on the very back of the foot running up toward the leg, is a very strong, fibrous cord. This is the Achilles' tendon.

3. Mark an X with your felt-tip pen on the very back side of this tendon at about the level of the ankle.

4. With your feet totally relaxed, ask your assistant to place the fingers of one hand on the ball of the foot to be tested and press upward with gentle to moderate pressure. Your tendency will be to help your assistant by lifting your foot, but resist this. Try to relax and, if anything, press down ever so slightly rather than lifting your foot.

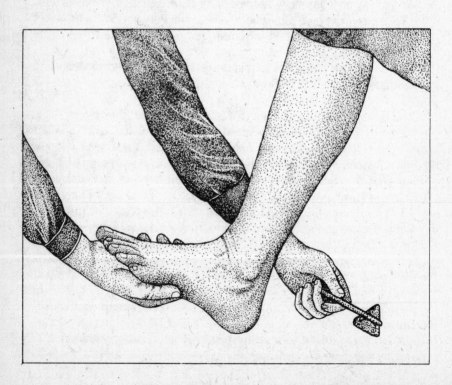

5. Now your assistant should strike your Achilles' tendon with the reflex hammer. It takes a moderately hard tap to elicit a response; you can't be too gentle, but neither do you want to deliver a damaging blow. The examiner should practice tapping his own Achilles' tendon first to get the feel of the test.

6. In most people, if the test is done correctly, the foot should jerk downward. Do the test several times until you get a consistent jerk with each foot. As with the knees, the ankle-jerk reflex should be equal on both feet.

Another reflex which can easily be tested is the arm-jerk or biceps reflex. The biceps is the big muscle which lies on the front part of the upper arm. The biceps tendon passes right down the center of the inside of the elbow.

Testing the Biceps Reflex

1. To locate the biceps tendon, first locate with your fingers the two bony prominences on either side of the arm at the elbow joint. About halfway between these two bony prominences, on the front of the arm, is the biceps tendon. Flex your biceps muscle and you will feel this tendon tighten.

2. Mark an X with your felt-tip pen right over this tendon in the little cup which forms when the arm bends.

3. Now ask your assistant to hold your elbow with his or her hand in such a way that the thumb presses gently on the tendon right where you have made the mark. Your hand should rest in a relaxed fashion on your assistant's forearm. It is important that your assistant support your arm in such a way that it can be totally relaxed.

4. Once your assistant has a firm hold of your upper arm with the thumb on the mark, he or she strikes the thumb pressing against the tendon sharply with the reflex hammer. A right-handed assistant would hold the arm to be tested with the left hand and use the little hammer with the right. A left-handed assistant would do the reverse.

5. The examiner should feel the tendon tighten under the thumb an instant after the thumb is struck. Your arm may also give a little jerk. Again, both sides should be tested and response should be approximately equal.

Tendon reflexes are an important part of a neurological examination because they help the doctor decide whether an existing problem stems from the brain, the spinal cord, or the peripheral nerves. A lesion of a peripheral nerve or certain parts of the spinal cord, for instance, results in a diminished reflex response, whereas damage to other parts of the spinal cord or the brain results in an increased reflex response. As stressed above, the equality of the reflexes on the two sides is the most important judgment to be made. Reflexes which are equal from side to side but apparently more brisk in the legs than in the arms are usually not a cause for concern. Generally, it is only when the reflexes become unequal on the two sides that a medical option should be sought immediately.

An overall assessment of motor functioning can be made simply by observing the subject walking and running. Simple as they may seem, standing, walking, and running are the end product of a symphony of coordination involving nerve impulses going to and from the brain and proper muscle function. Just to maintain balance, your feet must signal their position to the brain, which then instructs the feet to make any necessary adjustments to keep from toppling over.

Observing Gait

Ask your assistant to watch while you walk, stop, turn suddenly, and walk in the other direction; then jog in place for a moment or two. You should walk with an entirely normal gait, you should turn promptly without staggering, and you should jog easily on your toes, taking the weight of your body comfortably and alternately with each foot.

Actually, you are probably a far more sensitive observer of your own gait than any examiner could be, and you will be aware of even slight abnormalities if they occur.

Mental Functioning.   Finally, the last phase of a neurologic examination checks a person's general level of mental functioning. This is not an IQ test to find out how "smart" someone is; rather, it is a series of simple questions carefully designed to check memory of both the immediate and the distant past, awareness of the surrounding world, and the ability to perform abstract reasoning as demonstrated by simple arithmetic problems.

Checking General Mental Functioning

This test is much less formal than the others, in fact, except for the arithmetic, the entire test can be administered in the course of a casual conversation. You need not ask the same questions as those suggested below, as long as you check both short- and long-term memory and verify an awareness of major current events.

1. *Checking short- and long-term memory.* Some questions you

might ask are: Who is the President of the United States? Who was President before him? What time of day is it? What day of the week is it? What is the date? Who won the Super Bowl (World Series, Stanley Cup, or other popular event) this year?

2. *Checking abstract reasoning.* Abstract reasoning is tested with an oral arithmetic quiz. The subject is usually asked to do simple, single-digit additions. If these are answered successfully, the subject is then asked to count to 33 by threes.

The most difficult arithmetic test used by neurologists is the series-7 test. In this test the subject is asked to subtract 7 from 100. He produces 93 and the examiner immediately asks him to subtract 7 from that answer. When he produces 86, the examiner again asks him to subtract 7 from the remainder. They continue until the examiner has been able to assess the subject's speed and capability.

There is no question that many people find this test difficult, and it is designed to be just that. The test is also somewhat stressful. Thus while many people do not perform the test either very accurately or very swiftly, it gives the examiner some idea of how the subject performs under slightly stressful conditions.

And that essentially concludes a basic neurologic examination. Bear in mind as you review your performance that, for all their seeming simplicity, neurologic tests are very tricky to interpret. A response which might be considered abnormal for most people might be a normal variation in the case of a particular individual. It takes years of training and experience and keen observation to pin down the root of a neurologic problem. So these tests are not intended to be diagnostic of any disease or ailment. If you can get them to work for you, they are good indications that all is well. And no one is in a better position to detect slight abnormalities than you are yourself. Any unusual findings you uncover as a result of the tests in this chapter can be brought to the attention of a specialist that much earlier, and that can be important.

CHAPTER 4

TESTING URINE AND
THE URINARY SYSTEM

Urination is one of the most familiar body functions, but one that still isn't discussed much in polite company, in spite of liberated attitudes in other areas. Viewed with repugnance at best, the humble urinary system is taken for granted when it works, and cursed when it doesn't. Like Rodney Dangerfield, it just don't get no respect! Moreover, since the end of the system shares space with the genitals, disorders of the two systems are sometimes related and sometimes confused. Women, especially, tend to confuse vaginal and urethral functions and symptoms, simply because of their physical proximity and obscured location.

Unhappily, disorders of the urinary system are often fretted over in private with a stoic fortitude that is quite unnecessary, because the urinary system signals its afflictions in a variety of ways that can be measured and tested with just a little attention and respect on our part. You can set your mind at ease, or at least ascertain the nature of your ailment, with some of the simple yet revealing tests in this chapter.

Urination is one of the ways that waste is removed from our system. The parts of the body which are involved in this process are the kidneys, the bladder and the tubes which connect them, as well as the tube from the bladder to the outside of the body. Each kidney is connected to the bladder by a ureter. The tube to the outside world is called the urethra. This system is called the urinary tract, and it is the same in both men and women. The only difference is in the length of the urethra. The tube is shorter in women and this is one reason women seem to suffer from bladder and kidney infections more often than men do. Men have their own problems, however, because their urethra is partially surrounded by a structure known as the prostate gland. This is not a part of the urinary system, but sometimes the prostate becomes enlarged and makes the passage of urine out of the bladder difficult. The prostate gland itself is discussed in the chapter dealing with the reproductive system.

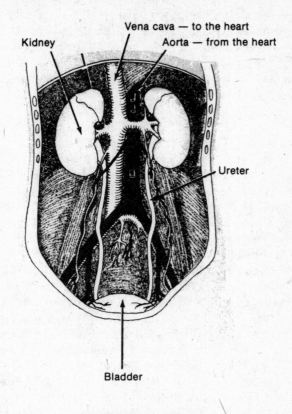

The Urinary Organs

KIDNEY PAIN AND KIDNEY STONES

The kidneys are located in the back of the body on either side of the spinal column. You can find the area where your kidneys are located by feeling for the edge of the lowest rib, just to the side of the spine. This point is known as the costophrenic angle. The prefix *costo* refers to the ribs; *phrenic* refers to the diaphragm. The costophrenic angle, then, is the corner formed by ribs and diaphragm. Some kidney diseases will cause pain in this area.

Testing for Kidney Pain

A simple test you can do for kidney disease is to make a fist and reach back and give yourself a few blows in the costophrenic angle. Just a good sharp rap will do; don't try deliberately to make it hurt. If this blow causes pain, you may have kidney disease and you should see your doctor. And if this little test is positive, you probably experience pain in that area when you jump up and down or when you are bounced hard in your car as it hits a pothole or goes over railroad tracks. You need not have pain on both sides. Sometimes only one kidney is involved, and only that one hurts.

Cuts and bruises of the kidney resulting from automobile or other accidents, or athletic injuries, may also cause pain. Many serious kidney disorders are painless, however, so the absence of costophrenic angle pain does not mean that you are necessarily free of kidney disease. But if you do have pain in the costophrenic angle, this is very suggestive of a kidney disorder and you should have it looked into at once by your doctor. One caution: The back is heavy with muscles at this point, so don't confuse a muscle ache with the sharper pain originating in the kidneys.

Two of the things most likely to cause kidney pain are kidney infections and kidney stones. Kidney infections are usually diagnosed through urine tests. Several of these tests you can do yourself and they are described later in this chapter. Some kidney stones are diagnosed entirely on the basis of a patient's clinical condition while others may be clearly seen on X rays. If your doctor suspects a kidney stone, he will probably take an X ray. Only those stones which contain calcium, however, will show up on X rays. Other stones, made of organic substances, cannot be seen with X rays.

Kidney stones are a perplexing topic and many times doctors will not be able to determine exactly why an individual forms kidney stones. They just seem to happen. These stones form in the part of the kidney where the urine collects before running down the ureter. They are made of chemicals which, for some reason, do not stay in solution in the urine but precipitate out as crystals in the same way that sugar crystals sometimes form on the bottom of a maple-syrup can.

In most instances, small stones pass through the ureter into the bladder and out the urethra. The pain occurs as the stone passes down the ureter, and it is usually described as intense and agonizing. It can feel like an acute cramp that begins in the side or back and moves toward the genital region and inner thigh. The pain may last for several minutes or several hours. Women who have experienced both childbirth and kidney stones report that the pain of a kidney stone far exceeds the pain of childbirth. Other studies of relative pain intensity also give kidney stones a high rating.

Once the kidney stone gets out of the ureter and into the bladder, the pain usually stops quite suddenly. The stone, however, may remain in the bladder anywhere from a few minutes to a few days. While the stone is in your bladder, you almost constantly have the urge to urinate and you find yourself going to the bathroom frequently and passing very small amounts of urine. This urge to go to the bathroom is also associated with infections. But if it occurs after a bout of super-intense pain in the back, it is likely that it is a kidney stone.

Looking for Kidney Stones

When the presence of kidney stones is suspected, it is a good idea to pass all of your urine into a container and then filter it through an old sheet or some other kind of cloth which will let water pass through easily. Cheesecloth is too coarse. Some stones are so small that they will go through the mesh of the cheesecloth. Hopefully, you will find the stone. Sometimes it is no larger than the head of a common pin, and it is rarely as large as the knob on the end of a hatpin. If you find the stone, be sure to save it and take it to your doctor. Laboratory analysis of the stone will help in determining the best way to prevent recurrence of this very painful problem.

Doctors use three basic methods for diagnosing kidney disorders. The first requires either X rays or isotopic scanning techniques. The most common of these is the plain X ray film and the intravenous pyelogram. The intravenous pyelogram (or IVP) is a test in which a dye is injected into your veins. This dye concentrates in the kidneys and shows up when an X ray is taken. The IVP test is very useful for diagnosing many types of kidney disease, but it is obviously not something you can do for yourself. The other two methods are blood tests and urine tests. Blood tests are also beyond the capabilities of most homes, but there are a number of useful urine tests which give a great deal of information and are easy to do yourself.

FLUID INTAKE-OUTPUT AND SUGAR TESTS

Sometimes abnormalities found in urine tests indicate a disease process outside of the urinary system. One such disease is diabetes. There are actually two kinds of diabetes. The common kind is called diabetes mellitus and is caused by a disorder of the insulin-secreting cells of the pancreas. No one knows precisely why this disease occurs. It may begin any time from early childhood to late in adult life. Occasionally it is inherited from parents, but most often no clear-cut family history can be found. Recent evidence indicates that some cases of diabetes may be a late consequence of a viral illness such as mumps.

The less common form of diabetes is called diabetes insipidus. This is a fairly unusual condition and results from a disorder of the pituitary gland. This is an organ about the size of a large pea and is found in the base of the skull.

In their earliest stages, both kinds of diabetes cause one to pass relatively large volumes of urine. The simple measurement of urine volume is, therefore, a useful test. To have any real meaning, however, total fluid *intake* and total urine *output* must be measured during the same 24-hour period. You usually begin in the morning.

Checking 24-hour Fluid Intake and Output

1. First thing in the morning, go to the bathroom and pass the urine which has accumulated during the night. Flush this away as you normally do and note the time. Then, for the next 24 hours, collect, measure, and record the amount of all the urine that you pass. Men can urinate directly into a measuring cup set aside for the purpose, while women will probably find it more convenient to urinate into a larger receptacle and then transfer the contents.

2. At the end of 24 hours, pass whatever urine is in the bladder and add that to the total. This represents an accurate 24-hour collection of urine.

3. During the same 24-hour period, record the volume of all the fluids you drink—water, milk, coffee, beer, soup, or whatever. Under normal circumstances the total urine volume will be a bit larger than the total amount of fluid you drink because most foods have a relatively high water content and add to the urine load.

Additional water is passed as sweat, exhaled breath, and in your bowel movements. At average temperatures and humidity, however, the amount of water lost through the skin, exhaled breath, and feces does not change very much. Urine volume, on the other hand, varies considerably as the amount of fluid consumed changes. If an average person drinks an extra quart of fluid in a 24-hour period, the urine volume will also go up by about one quart.

People with uncontrolled diabetes drink large amounts of fluids and this is accompanied by an increased urine volume. Sometimes urine volumes as high as 6 quarts a day occur. People with severe uncontrolled diabetes have such a tremendous thirst that they find it almost impossible to limit their water intake, even for a test.

If, under normal conditions of temperature and humidity, you find that it is extremely difficult to limit your fluid intake to less than 1½ to 2 quarts per day, and that your urine output is more than 2 or 2½ quarts in the same 24-hour period, you should probably see your doctor. On the other hand, if you find that you pass an unusually large amount of urine after a session of beer drinking, this is, of course, a normal phenomenon.

Some people have become habitual water drinkers, beer drinkers, or coffee drinkers and regularly have large urine volumes. This does not mean they have diabetes. It simply means they have fallen into the habit of drinking unusually large amounts of liquids.

FOR YOUR PERSONAL HEALTH RECORD

1. Measure your 24-hour fluid intake and urine output. Record quantities. Check every six months.
2. Record drinking habits—for example, do you habitually drink a lot of coffee, tea, beer, soft drinks, soup, etc.? How much?

As mentioned before, there are two types of diabetes. The common one is called diabetes mellitus, and the rare one is diabetes insipidus. Diabetes has been recognized since the first century A.D. when it was described as the melting down of flesh and limbs to urine. The name diabetes is derived from the Greek word for siphon because of the large volume of urine and the large amount of drinking that characterize it. The term mellitus is derived from mellite, which is a preparation of honey. Thus, diabetes mellitus is a disease characterized by excessive drinking and large volumes of sweet urine.

Urine Sugar Tests

An important test for diabetes is the urine sugar test. This is easily done at home by several methods. One of the best tests for urine sugar is manufactured by the Ames Company and is called Clinitest.® Most drugstores sell this little kit which consists of a test tube, a dropper, a test tube holder, and a bottle of Clinitest tablets. An interpretation chart also comes with the kit.

The best time to take a urine sample is just after you wake up in the morning. The urine is relatively concentrated at this time and the presence of abnormal substances will be more readily apparent.

To perform a test, place 10 drops of water and 5 drops of urine in the test tube. The pill is then dropped into the tube and a short period of boiling follows. The tube becomes quite hot so be sure it is in its holder. When the boiling is over, the test can be interpreted. If the solution is blue, the test is negative; that is, no sugar is present in the urine. Colors varying from green to orange to brick red indicate increasing amounts of sugar in the urine.

While many doctors prefer the test-tube method, there are dip-and-read tests that are easier to handle. In these you dip a piece of special paper tape or a plastic stick into a sample of urine. Color changes indicate the presence of glucose (sugar) in the urine and color charts are provided with the kits for evaluation. These are sold under such names as Clinistix® and Diastix.®.

Most of these tests for urine sugar are fairly specific for a particular form of sugar called glucose. Regular table sugar is a different form called sucrose and this gives a negative reaction with all of the sugar test methods mentioned. When you eat ordinary table sugar, the body converts it into glucose and this is what comes out in the urine of diabetics. If you wish to test any of the urine testing methods to see what a positive reaction looks like, do not use table sugar. Instead, take a piece of boiled potato, chew it a bit, and place it in a glass or test tube. Mix in a little water and test. The color changes will indicate the presence of glucose.

TESTING FOR KETONES, ACIDITY, PROTEIN, BLOOD, BACTERIA, AND BILE IN THE URINE

A number of other substances may appear in the urine that are indications of problems in the urinary tract or elsewhere in the body. Dip-and-read tests have been developed to check urine for these various substances. Because of the multiple nature of the tests they are sold with such names as N-Multistix® and are available without a prescription. Instructions that come with the kits must be followed carefully and precisely, however, in order for them to yield accurate results. Not all brands of sticks perform all possible tests, so be sure that anything you buy includes the tests you want.

Ketones. Diabetics who are in very poor control or who have not yet been diagnosed as diabetics will often show some ketones in their urine along with the sugar. Ketones are chemical substances which result from the breakdown of fat. This is not fat that you eat, but fat which the body has stored and is then using up. So the presence of ketones in the urine indicates that stored fat is being used by the body.

Anyone who is in a starvation state, and is therefore mobilizing stored fat, will show ketones in the urine. When very small amounts of fat are mobilized, the body is able to handle the ketones. However, when larger amounts of fat are being used, the body's ability to handle ketones is exceeded and they appear in the urine.

Ketones in the urine do not necessarily indicate disease. Patients on rather restricted weight-reduction diets often have ketones in the urine. One of the popular weight-reduction diets asks the dieter to measure urine ketones and indicates that only a positive result is proof of strict adherence to the diet. Anyone, in fact, who is on a diet which is restrictive enough to cause a substantial amount of fat mobilization will have some measurable amount of ketones in the urine.

pH.   The pH is simply a measure of urine acidity. Seven is neutral; higher numbers are alkaline and lower numbers are acid. The pH of pure water is 7, and the fluids in body tissues stay close to a neutral pH 7. Gastric juice in the stomach, on the other hand, is a very acid pH of about 2. Normally the body produces mildly acidic urine and a reaction of around 6 is not unusual. Certain diets and metabolic conditions may lead to the production of alkaline urine. Therefore, the pH measurement in any random sample of urine has little meaning. But if the pH is above 7, in the alkaline range, every time the test is done, this may be cause for concern.

Patients with chronic urinary tract infections often have persistently alkaline urine. The bacteria in the urine cause this to happen. And since bacteria thrive in a slightly alkaline urine, patients with chronic urinary tract infections are often advised to drink liquids like cranberry juice which produce an acid reaction in the urine.

Protein (Albumin).   The presence of protein, also called albumin, in the urine may be a sign of serious kidney disease. A small amount of protein in the urine is normal in some people, but large quantities usually indicate kidney disease. People who spend nearly all of their working day on their feet, not moving around too much, sometimes have small amounts of protein in the urine. This is a normal phenomenon and is called orthostatic albuminuria. When the phenomenon was first described, streetcar conductors were often used as an example of the type of occupation that might give rise to orthostatic albuminuria. But now that example has to be replaced by a more contemporary figure. Perhaps someone who spends the day behind a supermarket checkout counter would be an appropriate choice.

Large amounts of protein in the urine may point to trouble, however. Children with a kidney condition called nephrosis often have large quantities of protein in their urine. Similarly, adults with various kinds of kidney disorders may have a significant quantity of protein present in the urine.

Another Test for Protein.   As mentioned earlier in this chapter, protein in the urine is conveniently measured using the dipstick test. But another way to test for protein in the urine is by boiling about half an ounce of urine in a glass test tube. If the urine becomes murky or cloudy, add 15 to 20 drops of vinegar and boil it again. If it remains cloudy, protein is present.

Boiling urine in a glass test tube requires some care. If it is heated too fast, it will boil over and make quite a smelly mess. Boiling is best accomplished with a gas rather than an electric stove. Heat the tube slowly and preferably not directly on the bottom. Lacking gas and a test tube, you can boil the urine in a pyrex custard cup on a medium electric stove setting.

FOR YOUR PERSONAL HEALTH RECORD

1. Test urine for sugar. Record positive (sugar *is* present) or negative (no sugar) results. See your doctor if there is a sign of sugar. Recheck every six months.
2. Test urine for protein (albumin), ketones, and pH level. Note if you are on a special diet or taking any kind of medicine regularly.

Blood in the Urine.   Normally, blood is not present in urine. If blood does appear in the urine, it can come from the kidneys, the bladder, or any of the tubes connecting the various parts of the system. Passage of a kidney stone is usually associated with very small amounts of blood that come from the stones scraping against the walls of the ureter. The amount of blood is so small, however, that can only be detected with dip-stick tests or by microscopic examination.

Blood may also appear after a traumatic event. A hard blow in the area of the kidneys may injure them. This can occur from a football injury, in a fight, in an automobile accident, or in a serious fall. Microscopic amounts of blood may appear after minor traumas, such as a blow received in a football game, and will usually disappear within a few hours. Large amounts of blood indicate serious trouble, though, and a physician's advice should be sought promptly.

Disorders of the bladder will often make themselves known with bloody urine. And various kinds of tumors, infections, and erosions will produce varying amounts of blood in the urine. So bloody urine should never be ignored.

Not all red urine, however, is bloody urine. The urine can be colored red by many pigments. Sometimes food coloring will be excreted in the urine and will color the urine red without any blood being present. Beets, for example, will color some people's urine red when eaten in sufficient quantities. When women pass a urine specimen while they are having their menstrual period, it is often contaminated with blood, but this is not blood from the urinary tract.

The Odor and Color of Urine.   The odor of urine may change markedly but it rarely has any medical significance. If there is an unusual odor about your urine, chances are it is related to some food you have eaten. The most striking example is asparagus. For many people, asparagus gives the urine a characteristically foul odor, while others may eat asparagus and have no noticeable change in their urine. Other substances also change the smell of urine, but to a lesser extent. In any event, none of these odors are anything to worry about, because except for a few rare diseases, the smell of urine is not related to any particular illness.

Unusual colors in the urine, on the other hand, may be more important. As we noted in the previous section, a red color—if it is blood and not food coloring—is cause for serious concern and must be evaluated professionally at once. Very dark yellow or orange urine may indicate that one of the bile pigments is present in the urine. This happens in conditions such as hepatitis, which causes yellow jaundice. Two tests are usually included in multiple dip-stick urine tests—a test for bilirubin and one for urobilinogen—that show if substantial amounts of bile products are present.

Very concentrated urine may also be fairly dark in color without being indicative of any disease. Urine frequently becomes concentrated in hot weather, for example, if your fluid intake is limited. Some drugs can cause urine to turn blue or other unusual colors, which can be frightening if you have not been forewarned. If a doctor has prescribed the drug you will probably be warned what to expect. If it happens after you take a nonprescription drug, read the directions on the package or consult the pharmacist.

In a few rare diseases the urine is dark brown when passed, or it turns to a dark color when standing exposed to light. If you become concerned about the color of your urine, consult a doctor.

Bacteria.   Of all the disorders which afflict the urinary system, infections are the most common. Urinary tract infections should not be ignored. Left untreated they can eventually lead to long-term compromise of kidney function.

A urinary tract infection occurs whenever bacteria find their way into the bladder. Urine normally contains no bacteria at all. Stool, from the bowel, on the other hand, is loaded with bacteria and it is not surprising that most urinary tract infections involve bacteria which come from the stools. Women get many more urinary tract infections than men because the urethra is much shorter and much more accessible to contamination by bacteria from the stool. Sex play involving both the anal and urethral openings as well as soiled underwear are common culprits in contamination of the urethra, so scrupulous cleanliness in these areas is important. Women should always wipe themselves from the front to the back after they have moved their bowels, because it is very easy to cause a urinary tract infection simply by wiping dirty toilet paper over the urethral opening.

Several methods are available for the detection of urinary tract infections. Whenever you have the urge to pass urine frequently but only produce a small amount, you should suspect you may have a urinary tract infection. Pain or burning when you pass urine is a sign of infection. Although it is not terribly common, "silent" urinary tract infections can also occur. They are "silent" because the patient has no symptoms and does not suspect anything is wrong. This is one of the reasons that a routine checkup usually includes an examination of the urine.

The best test for a urinary tract infection is the urine culture. This must be done in a laboratory equipped to grow bacteria. In this test, a small amount of urine is passed into a sterilized container after carefully cleansing the genitalia. Some of this urine is spread onto a culture plate and then incubated. If organisms grow, it is possible to identify them. It is also possible to test various antimicrobial medicines to find the most effective treatment.

There are also dip-and-read tests that you can use at home to detect the presence of bacteria in the urine. It is best to do this test on a first-morning sample of urine. This will be relatively concentrated because you will not have taken in any fluid for a few hours and the bacteria will have had a chance to grow in your bladder for most of the night. You want a clean urine specimen for this test.

Taking a Clean Urine Sample

To obtain a clean urine sample, you should have a sterilized, wide-mouth bottle ready. It is easy to sterilize the bottle. Just put it in a pot of boiling water for about five minutes. Boil the lid also if you plan to cover and save the sample to bring to your doctor.

Clean the area around the urethral opening well with warm water and soap. This is particularly important because you do not want to contaminate the urine specimen. Rinse thoroughly so that no soap lingers behind. Have the bottle ready, but pass a bit of urine into the toilet first before collecting the specimen in the bottle. This is a further step to help avoid contaminating the urine. You now have a clean, first-morning sample of urine.

If enough bacteria are present, the test will be positive. This test can come up negative, however, even in the presence of a urinary tract infection if there are relatively few bacteria in the sample you choose to test. That's why in clinics and hospitals where laboratory facilities are available the urine culture is the preferred method for testing for urinary tract infections.

The presence of white blood cells in the urine is a good indicator of infection. White blood cells are rarely present in normal urine, but they are almost always present when there is an infection. The main function of the white cells is to fight infection anywhere in the body. Whether the infection is on the skin where you can see it or in the bladder where it is hidden, white blood cells will be there to do the fighting. If enough white blood cells collect in one enclosed spot, we call this an abscess. The collection of white blood cells, bacteria, and tissue debris inside the abscess is called pus. When there is an infection somewhere in the urinary tract, chances are good that white blood cells will be present in the urine in relatively large numbers.

To detect white cells you must view them directly through a microscope. Even the small, fairly inexpensive microscopes available in hobby shops are adequate. A simple high-power lens is all that is required. To look for white blood cells in the urine, the urine must first be concentrated. There are often not enough cells in an infected sample so that they can be easily seen without first processing the urine.

White cells in urine can be concentrated in a simple device called a centrifuge. This is an instrument in which test tubes can be placed and spun at moderate speeds. This causes the cells to concentrate themselves in the bottom of the test tube. By using a little ingenuity, you can turn several home appliances into a centrifuge. A variable-speed electric drill, a mixer, and the family washing machine are all likely candidates to become a temporary centrifuge. Here is how you can use the spin-dry cycle of your washing machine.

Looking for White Blood Cells in the Urine

Drill a hole at an angle into a block of wood to hold a test tube. Obtain a test tube at a pharmacy or medical supply store, or use the tube that expensive cigars come in.

1. Fill the tube half full with urine.

2. It is a good idea to be certain that urine has an acid reaction before looking for white blood cells. Test the urine with a dip stick. If it does not test to pH 5 or lower (acid), add a few drops of vinegar until the reaction is acid. The reason for this is that there are certain chemicals which appear as fine particles in alkaline urine. If the urine is made acid with vinegar, these chemicals will go into complete solution and not be seen as particles which could be confused with cells.

3. Place the test tube of urine in the block of wood and set this in the washing machine so that the top of the tube points toward the hub at the center of the washing machine and the bottom of the tube rests near the outer edge of the spinning basket. Pack the whole thing into the basket of the washing machine with some damp towels so that the weight is evenly distributed and the block of wood will not shift around while it is spinning. Set the machine on "Spin" and spin for three to five minutes.

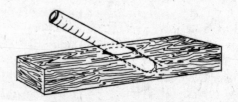

Looking for white blood cells.

4. When the spinning is complete, carefully remove the tube of urine and in one continuous motion pour the urine down the sink and bring the tube to an upright position again *before the last few drops fall out.* The solid particles, which include white cells, will be stuck to the bottom of the tube, concentrated out of the rest of the urine.

5. After you have poured out practically all of the urine, resuspend the residue in the bottom of the tube in the small amount of urine left by gently flicking the bottom of the tube with your finger. If any white cells are present, a white turbid suspension will result.

6. Place a drop of this suspension on a microscope slide, put a cover slip over the top, and view it under your microscope. (Follow the instructions for slide preparations that come with the microscope.)

7. White blood cells look like little black spheres. The illustration shows diagrammatically what white blood cells, red blood cells, and other types of suspended particles look like.

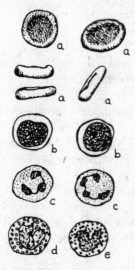

a = red blood cells
b, c, d & e = varieties of white blood cells

Most high school labs have microscopes you may be able to get permission to use, and many families have microscope hobbyists who can help. You may also find a centrifuge at many local high schools and colleges and a cooperative teacher who will help you perform your test.

Never let a urinary tract infection get a head start. Don't count on its "going away" because you drink a lot of liquids or because you use a patent diuretic medicine. Infections creep insidiously from one part of the system to another, and you want to avoid kidney involvement at all costs. Untreated kidney infections lasting even a week or less may cause serious permanent damage. So at the first sign of urinary tract problems, consult a doctor.

CHAPTER 5

TRACKING AND TESTING THE DIGESTIVE PROCESS

The digestive tract gets more media time than any other part of the body, and for people who manufacture things for the "tummy" and other parts of the alimentary canal, it's money well spent. The return in sales of laxatives, antacids, and other over-the-counter drugs for the gastrointestinal tract is approaching half a billion dollars. Still, most people know surprisingly little about this remarkable machinery that rumbles and grumbles while it does its essential job of feeding the body.

The best way to get acquainted with your digestive organs is through a laying on of hands, probing and pushing into your abdomen as your doctor does in the course of an examination. Under normal circumstances there's not much to feel except muscle and fat and an occasional slippery thing sliding under your fingers, which is exactly what the doctor feels when he presses and probes. But it's a good way to remember where everything is and it's important to know what your abdomen feels like when it's well so that you have a basis for comparison when you suspect something may be wrong.

LOCATING THE ORGANS OF THE DIGESTIVE SYSTEM

Except for the mouth and the esophagus—the tube leading from the mouth to the stomach—all of the organs involved in digestion are located in the abdominal cavity, in the lower part of the torso below the diaphragm. The diaphragm is the dome-shaped muscular partition that separates the organs of the chest cavity—the heart and lungs—from those in the abdominal cavity.

There are six organs in the abdominal cavity that work in the digestive process: the stomach, the liver, the gallbladder, the pancreas, and

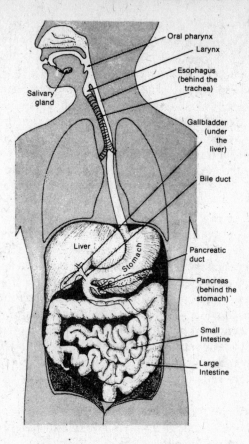

Organs of the Digestive System

about thirty feet of small and large intestines. This digestive machinery shares the abdomen with the spleen, kidneys, urinary bladder, and the reproductive organs in women, which makes for a somewhat crowded neighborhood, but each organ has its place and, generally speaking, they get along well together.

General Instructions for Palpating the Abdomen
You can feel your own abdomen or work with a partner. The directions given locate organs on *your own* right or left side. If you work with a partner, therefore, keep in mind where your partner's left and right sides are as you face one another.

1. Draw two imaginary lines through your navel—one vertically and one horizontally—to divide your abdomen into four quadrants. Lie comfortably on your back and relax your abdomen.

2. Place the flats of the fingers of your left hand on your abdomen. Press down on top of your left fingers with your right hand. Your right hand should apply the pressure while your left fingers do the feeling.

3. You can exert a good bit of pressure as you feel about, but use good sense. Your object is not to see if you can hurt yourself. If you intend to work with a partner, practice on yourself first, then make allowances for the size of your partner. You want to use much less pressure on a child than on a large, heavily muscled man.

The Liver and the Gallbladder.   The liver is a very large organ, much larger than most people think, and it has many functions in maintaining and monitoring body chemistry. One of its important functions is to produce bile, a chemical agent that helps break down fats so that they can be digested. Bile is pumped from the liver into the small intestine via the gallbladder, a small organ shaped like a tiny eggplant that hangs below the liver. Bile is stored in the gallbladder in concentrated form until it is needed. When fats enter the small intestine the gallbladder contracts and squirts out some bile. But bile can also go directly from the liver to the intestine, which is why you can get along very nicely without a gallbladder when it must be removed.

Locating the Liver and Gallbladder

1. Find the gristly bottom tip of your breastbone which feels like a little lump just before you get into the soft, fleshy part of the abdomen. This is called the xiphoid process. (Some people become alarmed the first time they find this bump, thinking it is some sort of tumor.) You are now on the vertical midline that you drew through the navel. The diaphragm is just above this point, so you are at the upper limit of the abdomen. Part of your liver is directly underneath.

2. From the xiphoid process, run your fingers down diagonally to the right along the bottom of the right rib cage. When you reach the bottom of your rib cage, where the last rib turns toward your back, you have finally reached the lower right limits of your liver. It is a huge organ; the largest in your body.

3. You have just traced the lower part of your liver. The rest lies tucked up under your right rib cage and its top rests against the diaphragm.

4. Go back to a point along the bottom of the rib cage that is about on a line drawn down from your right nipple. You are now in the vicinity of

where the gallbladder is hanging under the liver. You will not feel it unless it is giving you distress.

5. Lay the flats of the fingers of your left hand on your abdomen at this point with the index finger just rubbing against the rib cage. Apply pressure with your right hand on top of the left fingers.

6. Now, let the air out of your lungs, press down with your hand, and take a deep breath. As you breathe in, you may feel the edge of your liver pass under the fingers of your left hand either right under the rib cage or two to three finger widths below it. Whether or not you feel your liver depends on how you are built and how perceptive you are with your hands. But the real purpose of this examination is to get the hang of feeling your abdomen and to learn where your liver and gallbladder are.

The Stomach and the Esophagus.   The tough, cartilaginous tube that you can feel in the front part of your neck is the trachea, or windpipe, which carries air to the lungs. The esophagus, a muscular tube which carries food from the mouth to the stomach, is located directly behind the trachea and in front of the vertebrae in your neck, so it's quite inaccessible for feeling. The only time you become aware of the esophagus is when something very cold, very hot, or very lumpy seems to take its time traveling down into the stomach.

The esophagus is ten or twelve inches long in most adults and most of that length is in the throat and the chest. The esophagus pierces the diaphragm at about the level of the xiphoid process and makes a gentle turn to the left for about an inch and enters the stomach. Most stomachs are covered by a corner of the liver at this point.

Stomachs have roughly a J-shape but they can't be depended on to have precisely the same shape and location in everyone, so the following description may not be exactly right for you, though it is probably close.

Locating the Stomach

Contrary to common belief and erroneous diagrams shown on TV antacid commercials, the bulk of most stomachs lies just slightly left of center in the abdomen. Usually, not much more than a quarter of the stomach crosses the midline to the right where it meets the small intestine.

1. Place your fingers on the xiphoid process. This is about where the esophagus enters the stomach.

2. Draw a line from the xiphoid process on a slight downward slope

to a point on your left rib cage that is about two inches below your left nipple. This is the approximate location of the left limit of your stomach, which means that part of the stomach, like the liver, is nestled up under the dome-shaped diaphgram and is partially protected by the rib cage.

3. Drop down about two ribs and circle to the right across your abdomen almost, but not quite, to the point on your right rib cage where you poked about for your liver. This is the right lower limit of the stomach in most people, where it joins the small intestine. And both stomach and small intestine may be under the bottom edge of the liver at this point.

4. If you push in with your fingers after a large meal, you should feel more fullness discomfort in the area described than you will by pushing into the abdomen lower down, around the navel or below, for example. Keep in mind, however, that a few very normal stomachs do descend as low as the navel or further. What we have described are "average" stomachs.

Go back to the left rib cage for a moment, just under the left nipple. The spleen is tucked up in here between the stomach and the left side of the left rib cage. The spleen is not related to the digestive tract. It is a filter and storage center for blood cells. Once again, palpating around the stomach area and then under the left rib cage you are not likely to feel anything but soft, fleshy tissue. In some blood diseases or infections the spleen may become enlarged, in which case the tip of it may be felt around the left rib cage.

The Small Intestine.   Most of the abdominal cavity is filled with the small intestine. This mass of tubing, between twenty and thirty feet of it, begins at the bottom right end of the stomach and winds around and around until it ends in the large intestine on the lower right side of the abdomen. The reason for its great length is that most digestion and absorption of food takes place here, and a great deal of surface area is required.

Draw a line across the bottom edges of the rib cages, then go down to the pelvis on each side, and then across to the top of the urinary bladder—where the feeling of fullness is when you have to urinate. All of the area within these boundaries is filled with the small intestine. Pressing into this area should reveal no hard spots or any discomfort aside from what you would normally expect from being poked.

The Appendix and the Large Intestine.   The large intestine—called the colon—is the last part of the digestive tract. The residue of undigested food accumulates here and is made ready for evacuation by a bit more absorption of nutrients and the removal of water. The colon forms a sort of picture frame around the small intestine.

Tracing the Large Intestine

1. Find a spot on the vertical midline of the abdomen about halfway between the navel and the top of the urinary bladder. Now draw your fingers to the right until you meet the pelvis. The beginning of the large intestine is just about here, sitting in the inside hollow of the right pelvic bone.

2. Probe around a bit just under the edge of the bone and consider what goes on here. The small intestine is joined to the large intestine at this point. The large intestine—the colon—rises from this point to the bottom of the liver, and so this section is called the ascending colon. But there is also a small section of colon called the cecum that goes down an inch or so to a dead end. The appendix is attached to the cecum like a large, dangling worm that can be anywhere from two to six inches long. It extends inward, to the left a bit, from the cecum, and this is the site of appendicitis when it strikes.

3. Draw a line upward to where you felt for your liver. The ascending colon makes a right-angle turn here and goes to about the same site under the left rib cage. This section is called the transverse colon because it goes across.

4. Another right-angle turn takes the descending colon down to about the center of the left pelvis where it makes another sharp turn and goes a bit inward—this is now the sigmoid colon—which travels a short way to the rectum and so to the outside world.

Other Organs of the Abdomen.   The pancreas is the only other organ in the abdomen that is directly associated with the digestive process. It is buried deep in the abdomen, well hidden by the stomach and small intestine, and is even difficult to show in a diagram. One of its functions is to produce an important digestive enzyme which, like bile, is pumped into the small intestine.

The pancreas has a long tail that runs from the spleen in the upper left quadrant, under the stomach, and ends in a head that is tucked under one of the curves of the small intestine in the vicinity of the right rib cage. Because it is so inaccessible, trouble here is very hard to detect.

Kidneys, urinary bladder, ovaries, and uterus—all discussed in other parts of this book—complete the roll call of abdominal organs.

After you have explored your own and one or two other abdomens, you should have a pretty good idea of what an abdomen feels like and about where everything is. Probe every six months or so and in times of abdominal distress. If you feel pain or hard spots or lumpy matter anywhere, it should be reported to a doctor. Be sure, of course, that you don't create pain with overzealous probing. Have warm hands and probe deliberately. A light touch tickles. Remember, you will always find one little lump in the middle of the abdomen at the end of the breastbone. This is the xiphoid process that we've mentioned before, which countless people fear is an abnormal growth when they first discover it.

THE DIGESTION PROCESS

Chewing.   The first step in the digestion process is chewing. Chewing is important because it breaks food into small particles which can then be worked on by the various chemicals in the mouth, the stomach, and the small intestine. As you chew, saliva pours into the mouth from two little pimplelike outlets that are approximately in the center of your cheeks and can be seen rather easily in a simple inspection of the mouth, using a flashlight. Saliva wets down food, making it easier to swallow, and begins the digestive process by turning some starches into sugar.

Sometimes when certain kinds of foods—corn, for example—are not well chewed, they go right through the entire intestinal tract without being digested and are evacuated in the stools in almost the same condition as when they were eaten. Thorough chewing has many salutary effects: it aids digestion, it can help reduce indigestion, it helps in weight-loss programs because you feel full and satisfied sooner, and it can help reduce problems with gas.

The Esophagus and the Stomach.   When food is swallowed it moves to the stomach through the esophagus. Where the esophagus joins the stomach there is a circular muscle, the cardiac sphincter, that opens to let food into the stomach and then closes to keep it there. Beginning with the esophagus, food is moved along the entire alimentary canal (the digestive tract) by a series of wavelike contractions in the walls of the tubing. This is called peristalsis and it moves food in about the same way that you squeeze toothpaste through a tube.

Once in the stomach, food is treated with acid to break it up further and with enzymes which help prepare some of the nutrients for absorption in the small intestine. Some water, certain drugs, and alcohol are absorbed in the stomach, but this is not its primary function.

The Small Intestine.   When food is liquid enough or the pieces are small enough, they are squirted through the pyloric sphincter, another muscular gatekeeper, into the small intestine. The small intestine is thought of as being in three sections—the duodenum, the jejunum, and the ileum—although there is no really perceptible dividing point between one section and another.

At the beginning of the small intestine, the duodenum, bile is introduced from the liver via the gallbladder and a bile duct, enzymes arrive from the pancreas via the pancreatic duct, and other enzymes are produced by cells of the intestine. All of this chemical processing changes the composition of food to a form that can be absorbed and used by the body.

Food absorption requires a large surface, which is why the small intestine is so long. In addition, the walls of the intestine are lined with millions of finger-shaped projections called villi, which are so small that they are just barely visible to the unaided eye. These add tremendously to the absorption surface of the intestine. The villi are rich in capillaries—tiny blood vessels—and prepared nutrients from the intes-

Diagram of Villi of the Small Intestine

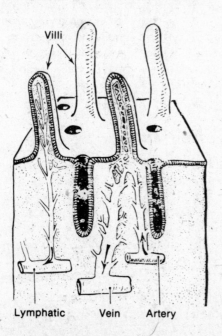

Villi

Lymphatic   Vein   Artery

tine pass into them. Larger blood vessels then carry the nutrients to the liver, where they are sorted and processed further before going on to the rest of the body.

The Colon, or Large Intestine.   You recall that the parts of the colon are the cecum—the dead-end section at the beginning with the appendix attached to it—the ascending colon, the transverse colon, the descending colon, the sigmoid colon, and the rectum.

There is yet another valve where the small intestine joins the large intestine that admits the residue of undigested food into the colon but allows nothing to flow back. A little bit more food value is extracted in the colon, but mostly water is absorbed there and the remaining material is compacted, mixed with a large number of bacteria and prepared for elimination.

Friendly bacteria which inhabit the colon perform vital functions such as producing some vitamins, fermenting undigested food, and combating harmful bacteria that may have been introduced into the colon. When, under abnormal circumstances, these friendly bacteria are killed off (during treatment with super-potent antibiotics, for example) diarrhea, cramps, and even intestinal bleeding may occur until the normal bacterial population can be restored.

Food residue is quite watery as it enters the ascending colon, but by the time it reaches the sigmoid colon it is fairly firm and compact—the very familiar feces. If it becomes too dry, constipation may result; not dry enough and you may have symptoms of diarrhea. Once or twice a day, or less frequently in some people, the compacted residue moves into the rectum where nerve endings signal a feeling of fullness. When you voluntarily relax the anal sphincter at the end of the rectum, the fecal material passes to the outside world.

LOOKING AND LISTENING

Get to know what your abdomen looks like. If your body is changing, all the doctor can see is what it looks like at the moment of the examination. It's helpful to know what your body was like before and how fast the change is occurring. If you have become paunchy, has the paunchiness occurred high, or low, or all over? What were your measurements six months ago, a year ago? Paunchiness may be the result of simple weight gain or loss of muscle tone—which is bad enough; but it can also result from organ enlargement or the accumulation of fluid, either condition being cause for serious concern. Isolated lumps, bumps, and swellings should always be viewed with suspicion, of course, and called to a doctor's attention.

FOR YOUR PERSONAL HEALTH RECORD

1. Using a tape measure, measure your girth in two places— just below the diaphragm (below the xiphoid process or tip of the breastbone), and just above the hipbones (the top points of the pelvis).
2. Record these measurements with the date they were made. Repeat the measurements every six months.

An interesting way to check the general level of function of your intestinal tract is to listen to your abdomen with your stethoscope.

Listening to the Abdomen

1. Place the stethoscope in your ears in the same way you did when listening to the heart. Place the end of the stethoscope over various areas of your abdomen.

2. You will hear a sort of gurgling sound which is not at all constant. Sometimes you hear nothing at all for a period of ten to fifteen seconds followed by a series of gurgles which last perhaps five seconds. The sound of the gurgles varies from a sort of low-pitched groan to a medium-pitched sloshing sound. These sounds differ slightly from one area of the abdomen to another.

3. Listen to various parts of your abdomen when you are feeling well and become familiar with normal gurgling. Try it just before, just after, and between meals because sounds will also vary depending on the extent of activity going on.

4. If a bowel obstruction occurs, the sounds change markedly. After a few hours all normal bowel sounds disappear. The abdomen becomes quiet except for high-pitched tinkling sounds. Or, the sounds are sometimes described as like water slowly dripping inside a sewer pipe—high-pitched and ringing in nature. Although the sounds are neither loud nor dramatic, they are very important and indicate the need for immediate medical treatment.

OBSERVING AND TRACKING PAIN, DISTRESS, BLEEDING, AND OTHER SYMPTOMS RELATED TO THE DIGESTIVE SYSTEM

When something goes wrong with the digestive system and related organs it will become manifest in a number of ways: pain, nausea, vomiting, diarrhea, weakness, dizziness, and sweating. Bleeding can occur at any point within the digestive tract and may or may not be noticed easily. When the liver and gallbladder are involved in a disorder, yellowing (jaundice) can appear in the skin or the whites of the eyes. Blurring of vision, muscle weakness and other signs that the nervous system has been affected may occur in cases of serious food poisoning.

Digestive upsets are so common and familiar that most people hate to make a fuss over an "upset stomach" or "a little indigestion" until the distress really becomes severe and can no longer be ignored. It is not at all easy to know when to worry about digestive upset or abdominal pain. But if you are familiar with the normal feel of your abdomen, if you know where the organs are located, and if you have become used to tracking the functioning of your body with a high degree of awareness, the decision-making can be done more intelligently. Here are some tips for tracking and observation.

Occasional Distress.   It is entirely possible to have quite uncomfortable abdominal pain which is of no serious medical consequence. This pain is usually of rather short duration and may be quite severe for a few minutes, disappear completely for a while, and then come back again. If this is an isolated and infrequent occurrence that disappears within 24 to 36 hours, there is probably no cause for concern. Persistent discomfort of this sort should, however, be investigated.

Severe and Continuous Pain.   Do not ignore stabbing or piercing acute pain or continuous pain of increasing intensity. Even a steady, dull ache can be significant if it is continuous. This sort of pain should be looked into by a physician without delay.

Indigestion.   This is a catchall, imprecise term for a wide variety of symptoms including different kinds of pain, nausea, "heartburn," and gas. It may be occasional and temporary, brought on by some sort of overindulgence or stress, or it may indicate something more serious. One clue is frequency of recurrence and the persistence of the distress. Track symptoms carefully: time and circumstances of onset, duration, suspect food eaten or drugs taken (including coffee, tobacco, and alchohol) and the precise location and nature of the distress. Then, if you have to report to a physician, you can do it accurately and intelligently.

A Word About Serious Illness.   While serious illness can occur quite suddenly—for example, a heart attack, or a bit less dramatically, appendicitis—more often serious disorders develop more gradually; they are more persistent and are accompanied by a more pervasive and continuous feeling of disability. Once again, *tracking* of signs and symptoms is important.

Pain of Appendicitis.   Appendicitis is very difficult to diagnose, even for a physician. If you suspect appendicitis, it should be reported to a physician at once for evaluation. Suspicious signs include: pain starting near the navel that migrates to the right lower quadrant and settles there; tenderness in the right lower quadrant on deep palpation and absence of similar tenderness on the left side; some degree of muscle spasm on the right side (this can be felt if you are familiar with your abdomen); low fever. Similar pain on the left side, if severe and persistent, may indicate diverticular disease—pouches forming on the descending colon—and must be checked by a physician.

Gallbladder Pain.   Gallbladder pain, which can be severe and knifelike, occurs in the upper right quadrant of the abdomen. Onset of pain may be associated with a fatty meal. It may last several hours and then gradually go away. Then, pain is likely to recur when another fatty meal is eaten. Severe knifelike pain should be investigated at once. The pain of gallbladder inflammation and heart attack can be confused and they occur with most frequency in people who are most susceptible through age and life style to both ailments.

Ulcer Pain.   Pain from an ulcer either in the stomach (peptic ulcer) or in the small intestine (duodenal ulcer) usually occurs high and in the middle of the abdomen. It is often so well localized that you can point to the exact spot where the pain is felt. Pain from an inflammation of the pancreas also occurs high and in the middle of the abdomen. Pain from any of these sources can be quite severe, burning, or gnawing, and may pierce through to the back. Ulcer pain can usually be associated with eating in the following way: pain may appear a few hours after a meal and then is relieved when something is eaten again. Incidentally, it should be kept in mind that ulcers are not uncommon in children and young adults as well as in older people.

Hemorrhoids.   Hemorrhoids consist of swollen veins in the area of the anal canal and sphincter. Hemorrhoids are classified as internal or external depending on whether they develop just inside or just outside the anal sphincter. There may be a mixture of both. They tend to hurt, itch, and bleed. Bleeding appears as bright red blood in the toilet or as spots of blood on toilet tissue. This bleeding is not dangerous and hemorrhoids do not degenerate into cancer. They should be checked in the course of regular examinations, however, and if they become too annoying they can be removed. But surgery for hermorrhoids, it should be noted, is being recommended less and less today as a good way to manage this problem.

Blood in Stools.   Black, tarry-looking stools may indicate bleeding somewhere in the digestive tract. This can be a symptom of any one of several serious ailments and should be investigated at once by a specialist. Small amounts of blood in stools may not be noticeable, and some outside factors that are harmless may cause the stools to look black. If you are suspicious, have a doctor check a sample of your stools, or there are kits available that enable you to do this test yourself. One such test is called Hematest® which tests for occult blood (hidden blood) in the stools.

Testing for Blood in the Stools

The Hematest® kit provides a good example of how these kits work. It consists of a bottle of reagent tablets and filter paper.

1. Smear a thin streak of feces on the filter paper.
2. Place a reagent tablet in the center of the specimen on the filter paper.
3. Place one drop of water on the tablet and allow 5 to 10 seconds for the water to penetrate the tablet. Then add a second drop so that the water runs down the side of the tablet onto the specimen and filter paper. Gently tap the side of the tablet once or twice to knock off water droplets from the top of the tablet.
4. Wait 2 minutes and observe the filter paper for the presence of blue color. A blue color is a positive reading indicating the presence of blood.

Instructions that come with the kits must be followed precisely. If you have eaten rare meat recently you may get a false positive result from the blood in the meat. If you have bleeding hemorrhoids or contaminate the sample with menstrual blood, you will also get a false positive result. On the other hand, if you are taking large amounts of vitamin C, you can get a false negative result. All of these instructions and cautions are included with the kits and they are simple to deal with. Several samples should be tested because blood does not disperse evenly in the feces. If you get positive results using one of these tests, further and more extensive tests should be carried out by a doctor at once.

Jaundice. Yellowing of the skin or of the whites of the eyes may accompany problems with either the liver or the gallbladder and should be given medical attention at once. Some people are plagued with gallstones that don't produce pain but do produce the yellowing effect of jaundice. The yellow pigment won't show up well in dark-complexioned people, of course, so your reliance in this case would be on checking the whites of the eyes. And since you would have a slight amount of pigment in the eye whites under normal circumstances, if you are dark-skinned you should notice and try to remember what your eyes look like when you are well.

The yellowing effect of jaundice is caused by bile backing up in the liver and entering the bloodstream. The kidneys extract the bile and it turns up in the urine. Bile products in the urine can be detected with a variety of dip-and-read urine tests that are available in most areas. Check with your pharmacist or a medical supply house. (See Chapter 4, "Testing Urine and the Urinary System.")

Again, instructions that come with the kits must be followed precisely. If you get positive results using one of these tests, further and more extensive tests should be carried out by a doctor at once.

Involvement of the Nervous System in Poisoning. Visual disturbances followed by muscle weakening and difficulty swallowing are symptoms of botulism, a particularly virulent food poisoning which results from eating improperly canned food. Symptoms can appear within a few hours or may take days to appear, by which time you may have lost track of what you have eaten. So you may not associate the cause with the effect easily. Food from cans that are bulging, especially noticeable on the ends of the can, or food from containers that explode when you open them, showering some of the contents about, should be avoided. (The explosion is an outward splashing, not the hiss or pop you hear when you open vacuum-sealed nuts or coffee).

Poison mushrooms and some kinds of tainted shellfish can also produce symptoms that indicate an effect on the nervous system. Report any such unusual symptoms to a doctor at once; don't wait for the "spell" to pass or go away. Delay can be fatal!

Questions You Should be Able to Answer.   When you have an abdominal pain or distress, observe it and track it closely; you may be able to provide vital information to your physician if it comes to that. When did the distress or pain begin? Where is the pain—exactly? Is the pain cramping, dull, sharp, piercing, continuous, intermittent? What other symptoms do you have with the distress? If there is vomiting, diarrhea, or constipation, be able to describe its onset, its appearance, and its frequency.

Palpation.   When you report abdominal distress to the doctor, he will probe your abdomen at once. If you have become accustomed to probing your own abdomen under normal circumstances, you will want to do this in times of distress. If you notice swellings or hard spots or enlargements or anything else that seems unusual, report this to the doctor. Sometimes muscle spasms come and go and will not be apparent when the doctor palpates your abdomen; but the information that you felt them can be helpful in making a diagnosis.

OBSERVING AND TRACKING BOWEL MOVEMENTS

One of the best tests of the gastrointestinal system is simple observation of your bowel movements for size and shape, color, consistency, frequency patterns, and changes that may occur in any of these things. Accurate information describing the past and present status of your bowel movements is a valuable diagnostic tool for your doctor when you complain of abdominal distress or when you are having a general health evaluation, and it is information only you can supply. Changes are especially important and the only way you can report changes accurately is to have a record that spans a period of time. Use a chart like the one below. Track your bowel movements and habits for a period of two weeks or so when you feel perfectly well. Track again when you change your diet for one reason or another. Track in times of distress. You will not track for two weeks, of course, in times of obvious distress or when something is plainly wrong—prolonged diarrhea or constipation, signs of bleeding—but any observation that you do have available will be important.

Date and Time	Description	Remarks

In the Description Column: Include such information as consistency of stool (wet, dry, hard, soft), color, size and shape, any strange or unusually foul odor, and some rough estimate of quantity—a lot or a little. More about these items in a minute.

In the Remarks Column: Anything should appear here that seems relevant to you—for example, a recent change in your diet, suspect foods recently eaten, tension or stress you may be experiencing, abdominal pain or distress, whether you have tested your stools for blood and what you have found, whether changes noticed are recent or long-standing. Record any laxatives, antacids, or other gut medicines you are using. Did you recently start taking any prescribed or nonprescribed medications, vitamins, or food supplements?

Generally speaking, people feel better and are more at ease when their bowels are moving regularly and easily. And thanks to commercial exhortations to "regularity," it is something most of us strive for without fully knowing what it is. Daily bowel movements at the same time each day are convenient and commendable but are not all that salutary if they are induced by laxatives on a regular basis. A laxative habit, in fact, while producing "regularity," can be harmful and of itself a sign that something is wrong.

No one pattern of bowel movements can be called "normal" for everyone. Some people have one bowel movement a day, some have two or more, and some people may normally skip a day, or even two, and then make it up with large quantities on another day. Track your own habits to determine what is normal for you. If you are not happy with the quality and quantity of your stools, try adding fiber to your diet—bran, nuts, raisins, fresh fruits, and vegetables, whole-wheat and bran supplemented breads—and see if it doesn't make a pleasing and dramatic difference.

Frequency of movements may change seasonally as your diet shifts to more fresh foods in the summer, or fewer fresh foods in winter. Travel, stress, and inconvenient or dirty toilet facilities can also affect the frequency of your bowel movements. So "regularity" does not tell nearly so much about the state of your digestive tract as the consistency, color, and any changes you may notice in the appearance of your stools.

Observing Bowel Movements

1. *Consistency.* Food residue is watery as it enters the ascending colon from the small intestine, but by the time the fecal material reaches the sigmoid colon and the rectum, most of the water has been absorbed; enough water is left, however, to allow easy passage of stools through the anal opening. If stools are dry and hard, they have spent too much time in the colon. If stools are loose and watery, they have been rushed through the colon too fast. If either condition persists, especially when accompanied by abdominal distress or upset, it should be looked into by a physician.

2. *Size and shape.* The size of stools depends on a person's size and the nature of one's diet. High-fiber diets produce larger, bulkier stools, which seems to be desirable. Something one inch or more in diameter is a nice size. Narrow, wormlike, or ribbon-shaped stools occur occasionally, but should they persist in this shape or if they are accompanied by increasing abdominal distress or upset, the condition should be reported to your doctor at once. It could indicate a partial blockage near the end of the colon.

3. *Color.* Medium brown seems to be the norm for most people. Those on vegetarian diets have lighter-colored stools while meat eaters' are darker. Various foods and medicines may create unusual colors: beets introduce red and may simulate bleeding; iron supplements and Pepto-Bismol make stools black. Black, tarry-looking stools indicate bleeding somewhere in the digestive tract and should be investigated at once. Gray or chalky stools are abnormal and should also be reported to a physician.

4. *Change.* Change in bowel habits is one of the warning signs of cancer. This is a prime reason for observing and tracking your bowel movements. Temporary or short-lived changes are inevitable, of course, as you eat different foods or experience stomach upsets. Changes may even be long-lasting if they are associated with a permanent change of diet—from low to high fiber, for example. It is persistent change in size, shape, consistency, color, or odor that has no apparent explanation or can't be easily related to a change in diet that you want to watch for.

TRACKING DIGESTIVE UPSETS
OF INDETERMINATE CAUSE

Many people endure chronic indigestion, constipation or diarrhea which persists, with no apparent reason, even after thorough medical evaluation has been done. Diagnoses are sometimes of "twentieth-century stomach," "irritable colon," or some other vagueness that means "there doesn't seem to be anything wrong organically so it must be something in your diet or stress or nervousness or something like that—." Sometimes when a doctor explains this and exhorts the patient to calm down, symptoms disappear.

In situations of unexplained and unexplainable distress, it may help to keep a diary of distressful episodes and see if a pattern emerges. Record the date and time, foods eaten, drugs being used (including tobacco and alcohol), whether you have been tense or nervous (record the circumstances), and make any comments that seem relevant.

Some people quickly discover this way that bouts of diarrhea quickly follow drinking milk or eating ice cream. Indigestion, constipation, or diarrhea may follow or precede going on trips, family quarrels, stress on the job. But if nothing else, you will amass a useful record for the doctor to analyze on your next visit.

Date	Time	Foods Eaten	Drugs Used	Stress or Emotional Upset	Comments

PINWORMS

Pinworms are tiny white worms which inhabit the lower end of the large bowel. Either adults or children may become infected with the worms, but children are generally the first in a family to get them. If you suspect your child has pinworms you should look carefully in the anal region either very late at night after the child has been asleep for several hours or very early in the morning before the child awakens. You may be able to actually see the tiny worms before they crawl back into the bowel through the anal sphincter after laying their eggs.

More often than not, however, the pinworms are not caught at the moment they have come out to lay eggs. The diagnosis of pinworm disease therefore rests on finding pinworm eggs. These are tiny little eggs which are microscopic in size. A pinworm egg test is relatively simple, but you must have a microscope to carry it out. Most home microscopes or those used in high school laboratories will do.

Testing for Pinworms

1. Take a piece of Scotch tape and blot it around the skin surrounding the child's anus first thing in the morning before the child gets out of bed.

2. Place the piece of Scotch tape on a microscope slide, sticky side down.

3. Examine the slide using the high-magnification lens on your microscope. The Scotch tape picks up a large number of dirt particles, loose skin cells, small hairs, and almost anything else which is loose in the area, including pinworm eggs. Pinworm eggs, however, are a very characteristic shape and once you see one there will be no doubt in your mind that you have found it. A pinworm egg is about the same oval shape as a hen's egg; it is clear and when viewed under the microscope a tiny worm can be seen folded up inside.

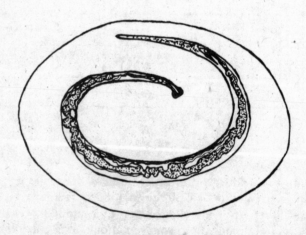

Pinworm Egg

For pinworms to grow, the egg must somehow be transmitted to the mouth of another person. This may at first seem difficult, but since eggs are only microscopic in size and very light, they can flow through the air attached to dust particles and can easily settle on food, dishes, and even someone's toothbrush.

If any member of the family contracts a pinworn infestation, the bed linen and pajamas for everyone should be washed simultaneously, there should be a general house cleaning, and everyone in the household should be simultaneously treated by a physician.

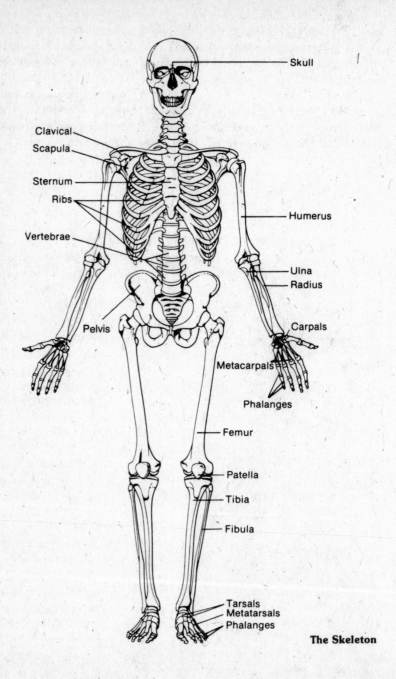

Skull

Clavical

Scapula

Sternum

Ribs

Vertebrae

Humerus

Ulna

Radius

Pelvis

Carpals

Metacarpals

Phalanges

Femur

Patella

Tibia

Fibula

Tarsals
Metatarsals
Phalanges

The Skeleton

CHAPTER 6

TESTS AND OBSERVATIONS OF BONES, MUSCLES, AND JOINTS

For most of us, the sum of our knowledge regarding the musculo-skeletal system is contained in that familiar anatomical ditty that goes, "the head bone's connected to the neck bone, the neck bone's connected to the shoulder bone . . .".

Actually, there's more to "dem dry bones" than is suggested in this song, of course. For one thing, our bones are neither dry nor old—they are composed of living tissues which are continually dissolving and regenerating in an unending process which completely replaces every bone cell in an active person's body over a seven-year period. Furthermore, the bones and joints that make up our skeleton are only half of the great articular system which gives the human body its form and allows it to take action. The other half consists of the muscles, tendons, and ligaments that hold the skeleton together and allow us to make precise and subtle movements.

While bones perform a number of valuable functions, their role in body movement is largely passive—that is, they do not act independently, but rather are acted upon by the muscles which control them. Skeletal muscles are attached to bones at either end of their length and are left unattached in the middle. The attachments are generally made across a joint with one end of the muscle attached to a bone on one side of the joint and the other end of the muscle attached along a bone on the other side of the joint.

Any individual muscle is able to do only two things—contract to make itself shorter, or relax. It does this in response to signals from the brain via the nerves that stream out from the spinal cord to the individual muscles. When a muscle contracts, one of the bones will move about the joint in the direction of the muscle pull. To get that bone back to its original position requires that the first muscle relax while

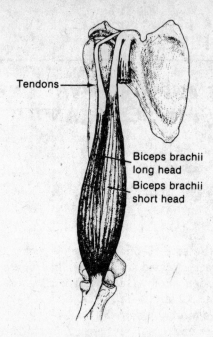

Tendons

Biceps brachii
long head
Biceps brachii
short head

Biceps Brachii Muscle, Upper Arm

another pulls from the opposite direction. Thus it takes a minimum of two muscles to move a bone about a joint and bring it back again.

In practice, however, a great many muscles are involved in moving any part of the body in any direction. It is this interaction of many muscles pulling in slightly different directions which allows the body to make subtle movements.

Consider your index finger, for example, and think of each muscle as a bundle of fibers which you can command to shorten or to relax. Now perform the following exercises with your index finger.

Observing Complex Musculo-Skeletal Movements

1. Hold your index finger out straight.
2. Bend just the middle joint without bending the end joint. This is a bit difficult but you can do it with a little practice.
3. Now bend the first two joints to curl your finger. Then bend all three finger joints as you do when you make a fist.
4. Holding the finger straight again, move only the third joint, the one where the finger joins the hand. Move the finger up and down and from side to side.

5. Flex just the middle joint and, keeping the finger bent, notice that you can still move your finger from side to side.

6. Finally, bend and unbend the finger joints and move your finger in a circle at the same time. This is the kind of finger dexterity you need for buttoning a coat, playing a musical instrument, or assembling the parts of anything from a model airplane to a computer.

Considering that at least two opposing bundles of muscle fibers are needed to make each movement, and considering that you have been moving only a single finger, you can get some idea of the tremendous number of muscles needed to give your entire body a full range of movement.

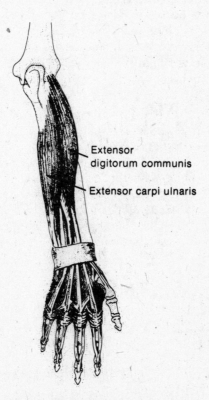

Extensor
digitorum communis

Extensor carpi ulnaris

Hand and Arm, Muscles and Tendons

While many of the muscles which provide body movement are located along the bones they control, others extend a rather long distance away. For instance, the small muscles which allow you to make finely adjusted finger movements are located along the finger bones. But the big muscles that give strength to your grip originate up in the forearm. You can sense this by making a fist and feeling the action of the various muscles in your forearm, in the heel of your hand, and in the sides of your hand as you clench and unclench your fist.

Muscles are attached to bones by stiff cords of fibrous tissue called tendons. Where the tendons pass over a joint they are enclosed in a tube called a tendon sheath. The inside of this sheath is very smooth and contains a small amount of slippery fluid that allows the tendon to glide smoothly over the joint. The joint itself is enclosed in a fibrous capsule which secretes a lubricating fluid that minimizes friction between the two bony surfaces that comprise the joint. And, finally, the bones themselves are connected to one another at the joints by ligaments. These dense, fibrous bands maintain the bones in their proper relationship to one another and give the joint strength and resistance to sideward movement. Without ligaments, joints would fall apart whenever the muscles began to pull.

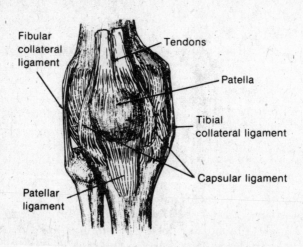

Ligaments and Tendons of the Knee Joints (Front view)

To review, then, the musculo-skeletal system comprises five major components:

1. the bones which give the body its general shape and structure;
2. the joints between the bones which allow the body to be mobile and flexible;
3. the muscles which, with the help of the nervous system, provide all body movements;
4. the tendons which attach muscles to bones; and
5. the ligaments, which hold adjacent bones together and keep the joints from separating.

There are a number of tests you can do yourself to check on the functioning of your musculo-skeletal system.

THE BONES

The bones of the body are hardly the inert girders that many people believe them to be. A typical long bone with the familiar, knobby ends consists of hard, compact bone on the outer surface, but spongy bone within and at either end. Bone marrow fills the hollow spaces in the spongy bone tissue and the narrow cavity that runs down the center of the bone shaft.

Bone tissue is composed of both organic and inorganic substances. The organic elements give bones flexibility and elasticity, while the inorganic constitutents give the bones hardness and rigidity. The bones of young children have a greater proportion of organic material than those of adults, and therefore are less brittle and more resistant to breaking.

Growth and elongation of the long bones in children occur at an area called the epiphyseal plate. This is simply a soft growth area at either end of the long bones where the shaft, or center section, flares out to form the joint end. When this soft growth area is replaced by bone, near the end of adolescence, further growth ceases.

Leg Lengths.   Most people's legs are very nearly equal in length. This is important because a difference of more than one-half inch can affect both your gait and your posture. When this happens, you must compensate for the short leg by placing abnormal demands on certain muscle groups in your body. In some people this can lead to chronic backaches and related problems.

A difference in leg lengths could be congenital, or it could be the result of abnormal bone growth following a fracture during the growth years. Or, one leg may *appear* to be shorter than the other as a result of a muscle abnormality. In any case, a marked difference in leg lengths should be brought to the attention of your doctor.

Checking for Equal Leg Length

The best way to check for equal leg length is to look for pelvic tilt. You can do this by looking at yourself in a full-length mirror. The test is best done naked. Stand up straight, facing the mirror, and place the thumb of each hand on the top of your pelvic (hip) bone. Check to make sure you are not standing at an angle but are facing the mirror directly. You should be able to draw an imaginary horizontal line between your two thumbs. If this imaginary line tilts up at all on one side, it may indicate that one leg is shorter than the other.

To be sure you are making your observations correctly, keep one foot absolutely flat on the ground and raise your other foot up on the toes a bit. You will notice that the thumb resting on that hip rises and falls as you raise and lower your foot. After raising and lowering your foot on both sides and watching your thumb rise and fall, again reexamine the relationship of your thumbs on both sides of your body. They should be exactly the same distance from the floor. If there seems to be a difference but you are not sure, enlist the aid of someone to measure the distance from thumb to floor with a tape measure.

Bone Tumors.   Tumors can arise in bone tissue as well as in other body organs. These abnormal growths may be either benign (noncancerous) or malignant (cancerous) and, if malignant, may have originated in the bone or spread there from some other cancerous site in the body. Although there is a rule of thumb that cancer in its early stages does not hurt, the opposite is usually true of bone cancers.

Recognizing a Bone Tumor

Bone tumors are most likely to appear in the long bones of the arms and legs.

A benign, or noncancerous, tumor usually presents itself as a slowly progressing lump or bone deformity. Typically, the affected person first notices a hard, immovable bony knob or mass beneath the skin that slowly increases in size. This kind of tumor commonly appears near the ends of the long bones—above and below the knees are common sites—and is generally not painful, though it does hurt if bumped or bruised. Although such tumors are not cancerous, they generally should be removed, and if you find such a lump or mass you should consult an orthopedic surgeon.

In contrast to benign tumors, malignant bone tumors are usually painful. Primary bone cancers are most common between the ages of ten and thirty and are unusual over the age of forty.

There is one type of bone cancer, however (actually a cancer of the cartilage rather than of the bone itself), which has its peak incidence in middle-aged and older people. Whereas bone cancers are most likely to strike the long bones of the arms and legs, cartilage cancers are usually found in the flat bones of the ribs and pelvis.

Bone Fractures.   Bone fractures, usually resulting from some kind of trauma, or injury, are among the most common bone disorders. A fracture is simply a break in the continuity of the bone. This break can take many forms ranging from a simple break to a segmental, or double, fracture or even an open fracture that protrudes through the skin.

The exact location and severity of a fracture is generally confirmed by X rays; in fact, some hairline fractures are virtually impossible to diagnose with certainty without X rays. There are, however, some characteristic signs and symptoms you can look for when you suspect a bone fracture.

Diagnosing a Fractured Limb

The most obvious symptoms of a fractured limb are pain and an inability to use the injured part. Immediately following the injury there may be some numbness, but this will gradually disappear and the pain will become more intense. Movement of the fractured limb usually causes the pain to increase dramatically. Pain generally increases in severity until the affected extremity has been immobilized by a cast or splint.

In addition, the following observations may help confirm your suspicions:

1. Tenderness at the fracture site.
2. Swelling at the fracture site.
3. Discoloration caused by bleeding into the tissue.
4. Muscle spasm. A muscle in spasm feels hard and tense.
5. A visible deformity in a limb such as angulation—that is, a bend at an unnatural angle. If you are uncertain whether such a deformity is present, compare the injured limb with the limb on the opposite side.
6. False motion or motion not at a joint.
7. Audible grinding of bony fragments on motion.

CAUTION: Do not try to induce false motion or audible grinding. These symptoms should only be observed incidentally while the affected limb is being examined or while the injured person is being moved. Testing for motion of the two bony fragments can cause further injury to blood vessels or nerves. Do not try to set a fractured limb yourself. Managing this kind of injury demands more training than you are likely to get from a first-aid manual.

Thus far we have assumed that the fracture involves either an arm or a leg. Other bones, of course, can also be fractured. Rib fractures, for instance, are fairly common and sometimes difficult to diagnose. A major crushing injury to the chest is obviously a medical emergency and you would have no difficulty in recognizing it as such. Lesser chest injuries, however, involving a simple, nondisplaced fracture of a single rib are usually much less apparent. Two tests are useful in diagnosing this kind of rib fracture.

Diagnosing a Simple Rib Fracture

First, simply observe the patient's breathing. A simple rib fracture often inhibits normal breathing. Someone with a fractured rib will tend to "splint" the injured side of the chest so that, when he or she breathes in, the injured side of the chest rises less than the normal, uninjured side.

A second test is to place one hand on the injured person's backbone and the other hand on the breastbone (sternum). Now press your hands together *gently,* as if attempting to press the breastbone toward the backbone. This would normally cause the average person little discomfort. If the subject has a fractured rib, however, this maneuver will cause a sharp pain at the fracture site.

Another common fracture involves the collarbone. The collarbone, or clavicle, is located just above the first rib, at the base of the neck. You have two collarbones, one on either side. This is a fairly common fracture site in children and teenagers and is usually the result of a fall or athletic injury. You can test for a fractured collarbone as follows.

Diagnosing a Fractured Collarbone

The collarbone extends from the sternum in the center of the chest outward to either shoulder. A fracture of this long, slender bone is indicated by pain in the shoulder at the time of the injury that is made worse by subsequent movements of the upper arm.

Given these symptoms, hold the upper arm on the affected side tightly against the chest wall, supported upward just a bit. If this position relieves the patient's discomfort somewhat, a fractured collarbone is the likely cause of distress.

Fractures of the back and neck pose a special problem because they can cause extensive and permanent nerve damage to the spinal cord. The immediate handling of people with such injuries is very important. If you suspect someone has injured his or her back or neck, check for loss of movement or numbness in the limbs. If the person is unable to move an arm or leg, or if a loss of sensation is apparent, do not attempt to move him yourself if anyone with experience in moving injured people is available within a few minutes' time. If you feel you must move someone with a suspected back injury, do not attempt to do this without some kind of a wide board. Slide the board under the injured person, changing his or her position as little as possible. Try to keep the patient as much as possible in the position he or she was found. Serious further damage can occur in attempts to move someone with a back or neck injury.

The other major body bones which are commonly fractured are the pelvis and the skull. These fractures can be extremely serious. A severe blow or injury to either of these areas should be seen by a doctor at once.

THE MUSCLES AND TENDONS

Muscles, as explained earlier in the chapter, move bones. They are attached to bones by stiff cords of fibrous tissue called tendons. Any single muscle can do only two things—contract and relax—which it does in response to signals sent by the brain via the nerves that stream out from the spinal cord to the individual muscles. Because of this close association between the nervous system and the muscles, it is often difficult to distinguish between disorders of the muscles and disorders of the nerves that serve them. A muscle may fail to work either because the nerve impulse to it is not being properly delivered, due to a nervous system disorder, or because the muscle itself is unable to respond to the nerve impulse. In such cases, even the experts must test carefully to determine where the fault lies.

Muscles and their tendons are also subject to a variety of common aches and pains which can be great or small and which may result from tension, unaccustomed or extraordinary use, fatigue, or injury. The causes of muscle and tendon hurts are usually obvious: overexertion without prior conditioning; a blow, a fall, a bad twist, or a pull; a tension-filled day where the neck, shoulder and back muscles seem to carry the weight of the world.

In most cases, muscle aches and pains of this sort, even when they are rather severe, are straightforward and relatively easy to deal with. Rest, aspirin, and reconditioning take care of most problems. Injuries to a tendon, on the other hand, or to the tissues where a tendon is attached to a bone, can be a more serious matter. But let's look first at signs of muscle disease.

Muscle Disease.   One of the earliest signs of a muscle disease is muscle weakness. Muscle weakness is a very gradual process which, for a long time, is most evident to the person affected. Generally, one group of muscles is affected more severely than others, and many times such disorders involve one side of the body and not the other. In such cases you can test for muscle weakness by comparing muscle size and strength bilaterally—that is, from side to side.

Comparing Bilateral Muscle Size

With the exception of your arm muscles, which may be slightly more developed on one side, depending on whether you are right-handed or left-handed, the skeletal muscles of your arms and legs should be approximately equal on either side.

To check for this, measure the circumference of both muscles at their widest points. A fabric tape measure used for sewing works well for this purpose. Be sure you are measuring the muscle at the same point on both sides. It's a good idea to first measure up or down from some bony prominence before measuring the circumference of the muscle. Compare your measurements; any difference greater than one-half inch may be abnormal.

Muscle disease affects muscle strength, too. Whether the muscle is at fault, or the nerves that serve it, a poorly functioning muscle will lose tone and then its strength over a period of time. You may be able to detect such a condition by comparing bilateral muscle strength.

Comparing Bilateral Muscle Strength

You can test bilateral muscle strength in your arms or legs by comparing the amount of resistance they offer when someone exerts force against them.

A test to help you spot muscle weakness in one leg is to lie on the floor on your stomach with your knees bent and your legs forming a 90 degree angle. Ask an assistant to grasp one ankle with both hands and try hard to bring the leg down to the floor while you use all your strength to resist. Now do this with the other leg. Your partner should find it equally difficult—or equally easy—to bring either leg to the floor. That is, resistance in both legs should be about the same.

You can compare muscle strength in your arms in a similar fashion. Stand facing your partner with your elbows at your sides and both hands held out in front of you, palms up. Ask your partner to place his or her hands, palms down, on yours and press down hard, as if trying to force your arms down to your sides, while you do your best to resist. Again your partner should meet with approximately equal resistance from both arms.

If one limb is markedly weaker than the other, it should be brought to the attention of your doctor.

Myasthenia Gravis.   Myasthenia gravis is a disorder of nerve and muscle function which, in its early stages, most commonly affects the muscles of the eyes, tongue, and the swallowing muscles. Women are affected about twice as frequently as men and most often between the ages of twenty and thirty. An early sign of myasthenia gravis is a drooping of one or both eyelids; the following test assesses the strength of these muscles.

Test for Myasthenia Gravis
A good test for myasthenia gravis is to sit comfortably in a chair with your head held in the normal position, facing straight ahead. Then, without tilting your head upward, stare at the ceiling for a period of two to three minutes. A normal person will be able to do this comfortably. Someone suffering from myasthenia gravis, however, will not be able to keep the eyelids open. Their eyelids will progressively droop until they cover most of the colored part of eye. After five to ten minutes' rest, strength will return to the eyelids, but on repeating the test the subject will again be unable to stare at the ceiling for a sustained period of time.

Muscle Spasm.   Leg cramps, a "stitch" in the side, swimmer's cramps, a stiff neck, or the pain that can "lock" your back as you bend over to tie your shoelace are all examples of muscle spasm. Muscle spasm is usually an indication that a muscle or the nerves serving it are in a state of irritation for some reason: the muscle may be fatigued from overuse; the oxygen supply to the muscle may be insufficient to support the muscle's activity; the muscle or its tendon may be injured; or a nerve serving the muscle may be injured or irritated.

A "slipped disc" between the vertebrae of the lower back can irritate a nerve, causing spasm in a thigh muscle or somewhere in the back. Shin splints, a common affliction among joggers, is actually a spasm of the muscles of the front lower leg. Cramps in the calves of the legs or in the stomach, the severe kind that cause numerous drowning fatalities, are muscle spasms caused by muscle fatigue or inadequate blood circulation that disrupts metabolism in the muscle cells. In a sense, muscle spasm is a painful signal to stop using muscles that are suffering stress of some kind.

Checking for Muscle Spasm

You can check for spasm by relaxing and then gently feeling the muscles in the affected area. If they are soft, they are not in spasm. If, on the other hand, the muscles feel hard and tense, spasm is probably present.

Tendinitis.   Tendons are the tough, fibrous cords that attach muscles to bones. When a particular muscle or muscle group is subjected to an abnormal stress—such as hitting a tennis ball or wielding an ax—the shock administered to the muscle terminates abruptly in the tendon. Too many such shocks irritate the tendon and the site on the bone where the tendon is attached. This can cause a variety of tissue damages ranging from surface irritation at the site of attachment to actual tears in the tendon or the muscle tissue. In extreme cases, a tendon can tear away completely, pulling with it a portion of the bone or joint covering to which it is attached. Depending upon the severity of the injury, treatment can involve simple surgery, immobilization in a cast, or just plain rest of the injured joint. Following recovery, the affected muscles will require rehabilitation in the form of special exercises to regain or, preferably, to exceed their former strength.

JOINTS AND LIGAMENTS

The joints of the body are the most complicated aspect of our musculo-skeletal system simply because they incorporate so many different components in their functioning. Muscles and tendons, bones and ligaments all come into play at the various joints to provide a wide range and variety of body movement.

As explained earlier, skeletal muscles are attached by fibrous tendons across joints so that when a muscle contracts, it can rotate a bone around the joint. This arrangement also helps to hold one bone in its proper relationship to its neighbor. But the main holding force is the ligaments. Ligaments are tough bands of tissue that bind adjacent bones together at the joint, forming a fibrous capsule lined with lubricating membranes (see the picture of the knee joint). In addition, joints are supplied with bursae (or bursas); these are flat, lubricating sacs inserted between two adjacent structures—tendon and bone, tendon and ligament—to prevent rubbing of these parts. And some joints, including the knee and the vertebrae, are also equipped with discs of tough, cartilaginous tissue that act as cushions, or shock absorbers, between the bones meeting at that joint.

Normally, our joints can take a lot of wear and tear and still function smoothly. Unusual stress on a particular joint, however, or a breakdown in any of its contributing structures, can unleash a wide array of miseries.

Arthritis.   The suffix *itis,* you may recall, means inflammation, and *arthron* is the Greek word for joint. Arthritis, then, is an inflammation of a joint. This general heading encompasses a wide range of joint disorders stemming from injuries, infections, or just simple wear and tear on the contacting joint surfaces. Its effects can vary from mildly annoying to virtually incapacitating, depending upon the nature and extent of the disease. Most cases of arthritis represent some form of either osteoarthritis or rheumatoid arthritis.

Osteoarthritis is the common arthritis of advancing age, generally making itself known after age fifty or later. Also called degenerative joint disease, this type of arthritis grows out of the accumulated effects of stress on a particular joint over a long period of time. The fingers and the weight-bearing joints such as the knees and hips are most commonly involved, and previous sports injuries to these joints make them particularly susceptible to osteoarthritis in later life.

Recognizing Osteoarthritis

A tentative diagnosis of osteoarthritis is indicated by some combination of the following symptoms and complaints:

- Aching pain in a weight-bearing joint (knee or hip) that is usually relieved by aspirin and a few minutes' rest.
- Morning stiffness upon arising that lasts a few minutes.
- Occasional swelling of an affected knee.
- Involvement of the fingers leading to deformities characterized by a knobby, twisted appearance. Knobs (Heberdine's nodes) sometimes appear at the base of the finger joints.

In contrast to osteoarthritis, which is localized in one or more specific joints, rheumatoid arthritis, or RA, is a systemic disease that is apt to make its victims feel sick all over as well as sick at a joint.

Typically, the onset of rheumatoid arthritis is manifested by general fatigue, weakness, a loss of appetite, a slight fever, and vaguely defined joint and muscle complaints which escalate into full-fledged infirmity. This crippling disease generally affects much younger people than degenerative joint disease—most often those between thirty and forty—and strikes women almost three times as frequently as men; and there is a variety of RA which affects children.

Recognizing Rheumatoid Arthritis
Rheumatoid arthritis can be distinguished from osteoarthritis by the following characteristics:

- Swollen, inflamed joints in the hands, feet, wrists, knees, elbows, or ankles.
- Reddened skin over the affected joints.
- Morning stiffness lasting an hour or more.
- Bilateral involvement—that is, the same joint is affected on both sides of the body.
- Muscle weakness and atrophy in the affected area.

The cause of rheumatoid arthritis is unknown and aspirin is the best drug for its treatment. Large doses of aspirin must be used, however, and should be taken under the direction and observation of a physician.

Joint Injuries.   There are miscellaneous sports-related injuries to the joints known variously as tennis elbow, surfer's knee, bowler's hip, thrower's shoulder, skier's heel, skater's ankles, and so on. Actually, while certain sports do tend to produce characteristic injuries, you can also get tennis elbow from chopping wood, surfer's knee from scrubbing floors, and any of these other conditions simply by abusing a joint with prolonged and unaccustomed use.

Their symptoms are pretty much the same—pain, inflammation, and some degree of incapacitation of the affected joint. The pain alone will probably be enough to send you to the doctor, and it's just as well because injuries to structures supporting a joint can plague you in years to come if not managed correctly to begin with.

Most sports-related injuries represent some form of tendinitis, bursitis, torn ligaments, or some combination thereof. You cannot diagnose the exact nature and extent of a joint injury yourself. But it helps to know what your doctor is talking about when he delivers the verdict. Here, then, are capsule descriptions of two of the most common joint injuries.

Bursitis.   Bursitis is often a byproduct of tendinitis, which we discussed earlier, and is usually the result of overexertion by the weekend athlete. Bursae are small sacs of lubricating fluid found wherever friction occurs between adjacent structures, such as between muscle and bone, tendon and bone, or tendon and ligament. Their purpose is to prevent adjacent structures from rubbing on one another and interfering with the smooth operation of a joint.

Under normal conditions, the bursae function nicely. Repeated abnormal stresses at a joint, however, can irritate a bursa. When this happens, the bursa responds by increasing its production of fluid, causing the sac to swell. Since there is no extra space in the joint to accommodate this swelling, the swollen and inflamed bursa impinges on nearby structures. This condition is known as bursitis. It can be extremely painful and is most apt to occur in the shoulder or hip. Treatment consists chiefly of rest.

Torn Ligaments.   Ligaments are dense, stiff bands of fibrous tissue which attach one bone to another at the joint and hold them together in their proper relationship. Without the necessary complement of ligaments to hold our joints in check, the bones would slide out of alignment. These should not be confused with the tendons which attach muscles to the bones *across* a joint.

Ligament tissue possesses a certain degree of elasticity endowing our joints with flexibility. Their elasticity is limited, however, and a severe blow or injury at a joint can tear some or all of the fibers that make up the ligament. This is what is called a torn or ruptured ligament or, simply, a sprain.

The most common sprains involve the ankle, as when you come down on the outside of your foot while running so that the foot turns inward under the ankle, or when a sudden force is applied to the outside of your knee, as might occur in a football tackle. Contrary to popular belief, a torn ligament is often *more* serious than a fracture and, if not managed correctly to begin with, it can result in chronic instability of the affected joint (trick knee, skater's ankle) plus further complications.

Since the symptoms of a pulled or torn tendon and a torn ligament are much the same, and since both are serious and potentially disabling, no assumptions should be made about an injured joint and no treatment should be undertaken without a careful examination by a physician.

UNDERSTANDING YOUR BACK

So far, our discussion of the bone, muscle, and joint disorders that can afflict the musculo-skeletal system has excluded mention of the back, but not because our backs are immune to trouble. In fact, quite the opposite is true—the back is prone to such an array of miseries that it deserves a section all its own.

Your back is one of the most vulnerable regions of your musculo-skeletal system. Not only does it have a large number of moving parts—there are 26 separate bones in the vertebral column alone—but the backbone is dependent upon an intricate support structure comprising muscles, tendons, ligaments, and cartilage. Working together, they can bestow on us the flexibility of a gymnast. Let one element go awry, however, and you may feel its repercussions, literally, right down to your toes.

The central feature of the back is, of course, the vertebral column or spine. This is a flexible column constructed of 24 separate vertebrae plus the sacrum and the coccyx—the last vestige of our ancestors' tails.

The vertebrae are divided into three groups. Starting from the neck down, the first seven are known as the cervical vertebrae. These are capable of an extraordinary range of movement allowing you to rotate your head from side to side and up and down. The next twelve are the thoracic, or chest, vertebrae, to which the ribs are attached. The brunt of the upper body's weight is borne by the last five, the lumbar vertebrae, and it is in this region that most back ailments are centered.

A typical vertebra consists of a round, flat bone and a pair of bony arches which meet to form a circular enclosure at one end. Three bony spurs project off this end of the vertebra, and you can feel the middle one, called the spinous process, as one of the bony bumps going down your back. When the individual vertebrae are stacked one on top of another, the circular enclosures form a canal down the vertebral column. This vertebral canal is the bony fortress which houses the spinal cord linking the brain with the rest of the body. The nerves of the spinal cord branch out to different parts of the body through openings in the vertebrae.

In between the vertebrae are those much maligned intervertebral discs, which are simply cartilage—walled capsules containing a resilient, jellylike substance. These discs act as shock absorbers, cushioning the vertebrae from direct impact with one another.

Each vertebra is connected to the one above and below by ligaments which serve the same purpose here as they do at other joints—that is, they maintain adjacent bones in their proper relationship.

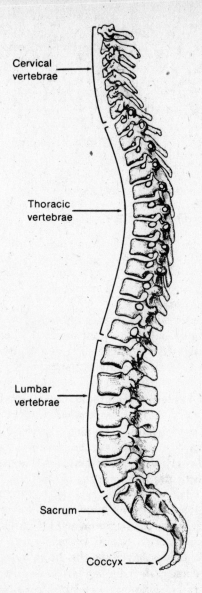

Cervical
vertebrae

Thoracic
vertebrae

Lumbar
vertebrae

Sacrum

Coccyx

Vertebral Column

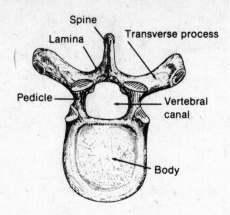

A Typical Vertebra Seen from Above

The vertebral column is held erect with the support of three basic muscle groups which, together, act as guy wires with each exerting the precise amount of pull needed to hold the spinal column erect. Many major muscle groups in the back, abdomen, hips, and thighs work with the back muscles to give the torso its mobility and lifting and pulling power.

The entire spinal column, then, is actually a series of joints, complete with muscles, tendons, and ligaments just like any other joint in the body. While the large number of joints allow us optimum flexibility, they also offer limitless possibilities for sprains, strains, aches, and related miseries of every kind. You should be able to diagnose some of these yourself or with the help of a friend.

Examining the Spine. The adult spinal column should be perfectly vertical, with a "lazy-S" curve when viewed from the side. This "lazy-S" describes the four natural curves in the back: the cervical curve of the neck curves in along the neck to the shoulders; the thoracic curve reverses the cervical curve, curving outward to just under the shoulders; next, the lumbar curve is an inward curve again at the small of the back just above the buttocks; and the sacral curve completes the "lazy-S" by curving outward at the bottom.

Lumbar Lordosis. A potentially troublesome posture defect exists when the lumbar curve, or lordosis, becomes exaggerated. Excessive lumbar lordosis, also called swayback, may be due to a genetic or organic defect in the spine, or may simply indicate a weakening in one of the muscle groups that support the back. If not corrected, this condition can lead to backaches and even disc problems later on.

Checking Your Lumbar Lordosis

You should be able to spot excessive lumbar lordosis in yourself by critically observing posture as viewed from the side using a full-length mirror, or in someone else by simply inspecting their posture from one side.

The lumbar curve, as explained above, is the inward curve of the spine in the small of the back just above the buttocks. Check to see that the abdomen does not jut out excessively in front, nor the pelvis in back. If you or your subject stands back against a wall, you should just barely be able to slip your hand into the space between your lower back and the wall. The greater the space between the lower back and the wall, the more pronounced is the lumbar curve.

If your posture shows an excessive lumbar curve, you should see your doctor for special exercises to correct this condition. Or, many good books about the back are available which tell you how to strengthen back, buttocks, and abdominal muscles and reduce lordosis to a minimum.

Scoliosis.   Whereas excessive lumbar lordosis is indicated by an exaggerated, inward curvature of the lumbar vertebrae, scoliosis is a side-to-side curvature of the spine. Normally, as mentioned earlier, the vertebrae should be stacked one on top of another in a perfectly vertical column. Any deviation of this column, either to the right or to the left, is abnormal, no matter how slight the sideward curvature may appear. This lateral curvature of the spine is called scoliosis and is most likely to develop in children between ten and fifteen, with the incidence being much higher in girls and more common around age twelve or thirteen. No one knows exactly why it happens.

If detected early, scoliosis can be corrected with the help of appropriate exercises and/or a remedial brace. The condition "sets," however, at about age seventeen, and treatment after that is likely to be more drastic and the final results less satisfactory. For this reason, it is critically important that young people be examined regularly throughout their adolescent years for indications of scoliosis.

Detecting Scoliosis

There are several checks you can make that may help you detect scoliosis.

The first test involves a critical inspection of the subject's spinal column. Have the subject stand up straight with his or her back bared to just below the waist. The little knobby protrusions running down the center of the back are the spinous processes of the individual vertebrae, as explained earlier. They should line up in a perfectly vertical column that does not deviate the least bit from side to side. Observe this column closely for signs of lateral curvature.

If you have any trouble locating the spinous processes, try this: Ask the subject to bend forward slightly from the waist; this will make the bony knobs more prominent. Then, using a black felt-tip pen, make a little dot on the skin directly over each spinous process (there are 24). When this is completed, have the subject again stand straight. The little dots should form an absolutely straight line up the back.

A dropped shoulder is another indication of scoliosis. Observe the subject standing up with his or her back to you, again bared to just below the waist. Check to see that one shoulder does not drop lower than the other. They should be equal.

A variation of this test is to have the subject stand with his or her feet slightly apart and bend forward slowly at the waist, letting the arms hang down in front and keeping the knees straight. As the upper body drops downward, watch closely from behind to see if one side of the torso is higher than the other at any time. Normally, both sides should remain equal.

Lastly, you may be able to detect scoliosis in its very early stages by recognizing an uneven development of the back muscles. Have the subject lie on the floor, stomach down, with hands behind the neck. Hold the subject's legs down and ask him or her to raise the upper body off the floor so that the chest just clears the floor, and hold this position for a moment or two. (*Caution:* Do not ask anyone who has been experiencing back trouble to arch his or her back in this way.) This position will exaggerate the muscles that run longitudinally along either side of the spine. Lay your hand, palm down, over the muscles first on one side of the spine and then the other. The muscles should be equally developed on both sides of the spine. Uneven development of the spine's extensor muscles may indicate incipient scoliosis.

Checking the Cervical Spine.　The cervical spine consists of the first seven vertebrae from the neck down. In addition to supporting the head, which is attached by ligaments to the top of the cervical spine, the cervical vertebrae permit the head to rotate 180 degrees laterally, and to look down at the ground and straight up. The nerves of the spinal cord that exit through openings in the cervical vertebrae serve the upper chest wall, the arms, and the hands. Pressure on these nerves, due to disc disease or arthritis, for example, can cause symptoms that mimic angina pectoris ("heart pain")—discomfort in the chest that radiates down one or both arms. You can differentiate between heart pain and pain originating in the cervical spine with the following test.

Checking the Cervical Spine

Abnormal sensations such as numbness, tightness, or tingling involving the upper chest wall, the arms, and the hands may be caused by a problem in the cervical spine.

To check for this, touch your chin to your chest. If this movement causes abnormal sensations in the upper chest, arms, or hands, and if tilting your head way back relieves the discomfort, you may have a problem with the cervical vertebrae. Now touch your chin to each shoulder and then each ear to your shoulder. If any of these movements reproduce your symptoms, the upper spine rather than the heart is the likely offender.

Slipped Disc.   One of the most troublesome of all back problems is the slipped disc. The spinal column, as you will recall, is made up of a series of small bones, the vertebrae, stacked one on top of the other. In between each vertebrae is a circular capsule—the disc—consisting of a resilient, cartilaginous shell and a pulpy, gellike center. If you can imagine a jellybean inside a tiny tire casing, the consistency of the layers might be about right. The discs function as shock absorbers between the vertebrae, expanding and compressing in various directions as you twist, bend, jump, and strain.

Healthy discs can take a lot of abuse. But a degenerated disc is a calamity waiting to happen. Doctors are not always clear as to why a disc degenerates. Age is one factor—as we grow older, the discs become less resilient. But then, young people suffer from slipped discs too. Poor muscle tone in one of the muscle groups that support the back certainly may be a contributing factor. Key muscles that aren't doing their job place abnormal strains on the spine and induce slight but potentially devastating changes in the relationship of the vertebrae, the discs, and their associated structures. And, of course, an accident or injury can damage a disc.

Whatever the underlying cause, the casing of a degenerated disc capsule eventually protrudes into the spinal canal, or even ruptures, allowing some of the pulpy center to ooze out. When the oozing material causes pressure on a nerve or nerves of the spinal column, this creates pain which sends your muscles into spasm and you to bed.

Fortunately, slipped discs are not nearly as common as simple muscle strain. Both of them can put you out of commission for considerable lengths of time and make you acutely miserable, but it is important to recognize a true slipped disc so that you do not further aggravate the condition with improper treatment. Exercises and certain chiropractic treatments which may relieve pain caused by sore or injured muscles may cause severe nerve injury where a disc is involved.

Since discs do not show up on standard X-rays, actual verification of a slipped disc is obtained by a myelogram. This is a special kind of X ray involving the injection of a dye into the spinal canal. But generally, slipped discs are first diagnosed symptomatically. Following are some simple tests you can do that may indicate the presence of a slipped disc. If your back problem seems to conform to this picture, you should consult an orthopedist or neurologist without delay.

Testing for a Slipped Disc

Slipped discs most commonly occur in the lumbar region comprising the lower five vertebrae that support the bulk of the body's weight. A slipped disc here almost invariably irritates one or the other of the sciatic nerves which run down the back of the legs. The following tests are designed to demonstrate, either directly or indirectly, this irritation of the sciatic nerve.

1. Leg Raise. Lie down on the floor on your back and, keeping your legs straight, raise first one leg and then the other off the floor as high as you comfortably can. Normally, you should be able to raise each leg about 90°, so that the bottom of your foot is facing the ceiling. If, however, you have a slipped disc, you will be unable to raise one leg more than 45 degrees or so from the floor without pain. If you encounter such pain, *do not* try to fight it and force your leg higher; this will only inflame the already irritated sciatic nerve.

2. Toe touch. Like the leg raise, this is another demonstration of sciatic nerve irritation. Standing with your legs straight, bend over and try to touch your toes with the tips of your fingers. An average person can get within a few inches of the floor or at least to the knees, whereas the victim of a slipped disc will most likely fall far short of even reaching the knees because of a painful pulling in the back of one leg. If such a person were to try to touch his or her toes one leg at a time, he or she would perform much better on one side than the other.

3. Testing for neurological changes. A long-standing disc problem

can result in varying degrees of neurological deterioration as indicated by weakness, numbness, tingling, or decreased reflexes in the affected leg, possibly as far down as the foot.

To check for this, refer to the chapter on the nervous system. Four tests here may be helpful to you in determining whether one leg has been affected by chronic disc disease. They are: "Testing Tactile Sensation," "Testing Superficial Pain Sensation" (you should be testing the feet and legs in both cases), "Testing the Knee-Jerk Reflex," and "Testing the Ankle-Jerk Reflex." The most important judgment to be made when carrying out these tests is equality of response—your reflexes should be equally strong in both legs, and both limbs should be equally sensitive to pinpricks and light touch sensations.

4. Testing for muscle weakness. A painful disc condition with sciatica can, over a period of time, result in a loss of muscle tone in the affected leg. To check for this, you should compare bilateral muscle size and strength in the calves or thighs, whichever seems to be affected by your ailment, using the muscle tests described earlier in this chapter.

Not every slipped-disc sufferer will exhibit all of the symptoms indicated by the above tests. But persistent backaches accompanied by pain in one buttock and down the leg, plus a positive response to any of the above tests, should be enough to send you to a specialist.

A Check List for Back Problems That Are About to Happen.   Some back problems result from a single accident, but most develop slowly over the years as a result of deterioration of muscles that support the back (back, hip, and abdominal muscles), and as a result of misusing and abusing the back. If you answer *yes* to three or more of the following questions, chances are good that if you don't already have back problems you soon will.

- When you stand naturally with your heels and shoulders against a wall, can you slip your clenched fist between the wall and the small of your back just above the buttocks? (This is too much lordosis and indicates poor posture.)
- Do you regularly sleep on your stomach or spend long periods of time lying on your stomach?
- Do you pick up items from the floor (even small ones) by bending forward from the waist without bending your knees?
- Do you bend forward from the hips with your knees stiff when you lift packages from the trunk of a car?

• Does your job require long hours of standing or sitting without adequate back support?
• Do you spend long hours in a chair where your upper legs slant downward from your hips to your knees?
• Do you frequently have to lift heavy items from a shelf or platform that is higher than your waist?
• Do you frequently have to lift a heavy object and twist your body to place the object somewhere?
• Are you more than ten pounds overweight?
• Do the minimal strength and flexibility tests at the end of this chapter. Did you fail any of them?
• Are your stomach muscles flabby and paunchy?
• Do you exercise less than twice a week?
• Do you engage in a sport (without prior back-muscle conditioning) that requires sudden and severe twisting of the torso (golf, tennis, football)?

Actually, even *one* yes answer represents an abuse of your back that can lead to back instability and consequent back ailments. If you have several yes answers you would do well to read one of the many "back" books available in most libraries. If you already have severe and chronic back problems, or if your back is frequently subjected to abuse, you should discuss corrective measures with an orthopedist or a neurologist.

TESTS FOR MINIMUM STRENGTH AND FLEXIBILITY

The ultimate test of the musculo-skeletal system is, of course, how well it serves you in your daily life. At the very least, your body should be strong enough to allow you to cope with normal demands likely to be put upon it. Unfortunately, even this modest goal is seldom realized. In fact, it has been estimated that more than half of all Americans— young and old—cannot meet even minimum standards of physical strength.

The following six tests were designed to determine the minimum physical strength and flexibility required for ordinary people in routine daily living. Known as the Kraus-Weber Tests for Minimum Strength and Flexibility, they provide a yardstick by which to assess the basic well-being of your musculo-skeletal system. The tests are simple, and are safe for healthy people of all ages. (If you are convalescing from an illness or if you suffer from back problems, you should not attempt these tests without first checking with your doctor.)

Kraus-Weber Tests for Minimum Strength and Flexibility

1. Lie down on the floor on your back with your hands on the floor, palms up, next to your neck. Keeping your legs straight, you should be able to raise them approximately ten inches off the floor and hold them there for ten seconds.

2. Lie down on your back with your feet tucked securely under a couch or chair, or ask someone to hold your feet down for you. Place your hands behind your neck. Keeping your hands straight, you should be able to roll up slowly and deliberately to a sitting position.

3. Lie down on the floor on your back, with your knees bent this time, and your feet secured under a couch or chair or held down by a partner, as above. Again, you should be able to roll to a sitting position.

4. Lie down on your stomach with a pillow placed under the pelvic area and your feet held down securely. With your hands behind your neck, raise your head and chest off the floor and hold this position for ten seconds. Do not overarch your back doing this—it is enough if the torso just clears the floor.

5. Lie face down on the floor, once again with a pillow under your pelvic area. You will need a partner to press down on your upper back in order to hold your chest to the floor. From this position you should be able to raise your legs off the floor, keeping them straight, and hold them there for ten seconds.

6. Finally, you should be able to bend over from the waist and, keeping your legs straight and feet together, touch your fingertips to the floor.

Simple as these tests may seem, it is amazing how many people cannot meet even these minimum standards of strength and flexibility. If you can't do any of these tests, you should seriously consider enrolling in a reputable fitness program. Getting into shape is easier than you think, and the benefits to your musculo-skeletal system and other body systems may well give you that extra measure of vitality you need to work and play as hard as you wish.

CHAPTER 7

TESTING THE EARS, NOSE, MOUTH, THROAT, AND NECK

The nose, mouth, and throat are essentially a single chamber divided by partitions at various places and at various angles. The ear is connected to this chamber via a little tube called the Eustachian tube which runs from the middle ear to the back of the throat. Because of these interconnecting passageways, an infection in one part of the chamber is easily spread to adjacent areas. That's why the common cold can affect you with a sore throat, a stuffy nose, and, if you blow too hard, an ear infection all at the same time.

There are a variety of tests you can perform to check the ears, nose, mouth, and throat. Most of them require a minimum of professional equipment, and some consist simply of knowing what to look for. You may find it worthwhile, however, to purchase an otoscope for your medical supplies kit, particularly if you or someone in your family has a history of ear infections.

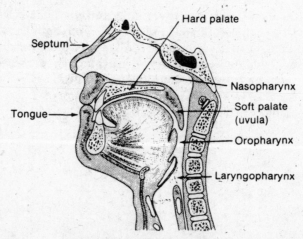

Mouth, Nose and Throat Chambers

An otoscope is a small, hand-held instrument which enables an examiner to peer into the external ear canal or nasal cavity. This can be a valuable aid in identifying abnormal conditions which require medical attention. The device consists of a little funnel which is placed in the ear or nose, a light arranged in such a way that it shines down the center of the funnel, and a lens which magnifies whatever there is to be seen at the far end of the funnel. A serviceable instrument suitable for home use can be purchased from medical supply houses starting at about $40, depending upon the brand and model.

Should you go shopping for an otoscope, you will likely be shown kits consisting of a handle containing batteries and a switch, interchangeable otoscope and ophthalmoscope heads, different size funnels for different size ear canals as well as for the broader nasal openings, and a handsome carrying case. The ophthalmoscope head is for

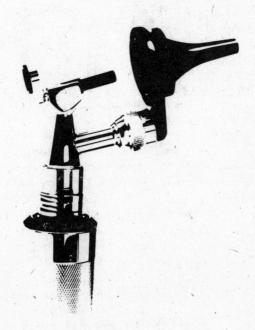

Otoscope

Courtesy of Welch Allyn, Inc.

looking into the eyes and from the point of view of the home observer, is not particularly useful. It takes a great deal of technical knowledge to understand what can be seen through an ophthalmoscope, and a fair amount of practice to even see anything at all. Since it is possible to purchase the component parts individually, you would be better advised to save your money on the ophthalmoscope head and the carrying case and buy only the handle, the otoscope head (some convert to a throat illuminator), and the assorted funnels.

THE EARS

Before actually examining the ear, it is helpful to understand how the ear is constructed and what you are likely to find when you go looking.

The ear is anatomically divided into three sections: the outer or external ear, the middle ear, and the inner ear.

The outer ear consists of a shell-like, cartilaginous flap that acts as a funnel, catching sounds and channeling them into the external auditory canal. This one-quarter-inch-wide canal runs a little more than an inch inside the head and is sealed off at its inner end by a cone-shaped membrane known as the eardrum. You should be able to see the eardrum using an otoscope by following the instructions presented further on in this chapter. This membrane, of course, effectively obstructs any view of the middle and inner ear.

The middle ear consists of a small cavity containing a chain of three minuscule bones called the anvil, the hammer, and the stirrup, because of their fanciful resemblance to these objects. One end of this chain—the hammer—makes contact with the eardrum, while the other end—the stirrup—communicates with the inner ear via an organ called the cochlea. The spiral-shaped cochlea is about a quarter-inch across at its base and contains the auditory nerve endings which transmit sound to the brain. The brain decodes the myriad sounds which are fed to it through the auditory nerve and converts them into meaningful messages. The cochlea together with the three semicircular canals, which help with balance, constitute the inner ear.

Because the middle ear is sealed in by the eardrum, air-pressure differences would build up within this cavity if it did not have some other connection to the outside world. This connection is provided by a slender tube called the Eustachian tube which extends from the middle ear into the throat. Its function is to equalize pressure on both sides of the eardrum. If the pressure on the outside of the eardrum changes for any reason, such as a loud noise, a change in atmospheric pressure, a ride in an elevator or an airplane, the pressure within the middle ear

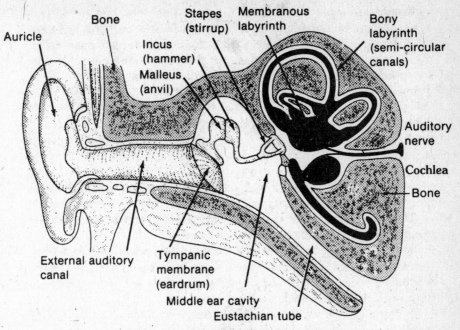

Right ear: External, Middle and Inner Parts

must adjust to that on the outside. If pressure equalization does not occur, we say that our ears are plugged up, and we cannot hear properly until they become unplugged. Most of us have experienced this feeling when riding on an airplane or driving in the mountains. In order to "unplug" our ears, we swallow. This action automatically opens the Eustachian tubes in the throat, thereby providing the middle ear with access to the outside world and a means of regulating air pressure on both sides of the eardrum.

A similar situation occurs when the middle ear becomes infected. The infection itself is usually not particularly painful. But when it clogs the slender Eustachian tubes leading down to the throat, pressure builds up in the middle ear producing a feeling of acute discomfort. A doctor may prescribe decongestant nose drops in treating a middle ear infection in order to bathe the ends of the Eustachian tubes, which come out in the upper part of the throat, with the decongestant solution. This helps them to open up and thereby release the pressure. Nose drops taken for this purpose must be administered with the head tipped sharply back so that the solution actually runs down into the throat.

Inspecting the External Ear Canal.   The only part of the ear available for direct inspection is the external or outer ear. This includes the external auditory canal and the eardrum itself. As noted earlier in this chapter, an otoscope is a valuable aid in examining the outer ear. If you have invested in an otoscope, here is how you use it.

Using an Otoscope

You cannot, of course, examine your own ear with an otoscope. You will have to look at someone else's ear and someone else will have to look at yours.

1. To use the otoscope, the subject should either be seated or lying down with the head resting comfortably against a pillow, a high-backed chair, or wall. The subject's head should be turned somewhat to bring the ear forward for easy examination.

2. First, brushing the hair out of the way, take hold of the rear cartilaginous flap of the outer ear between your thumb and forefinger and pull it firmly backward. This straightens out the ear canal, which is normally bent just a little.

3. Before you insert an otoscope in someone's ear, bear in mind that a careful examiner never pokes any kind of instrument into a body orifice without watching to see where the instrument is going. Always look into the otoscope as you perform your inspection. Never penetrate deeper without first making absolutely certain that you have a clear and unobstructed path.

4. Now, with the otoscope light switched on, insert the tip of the funnel just inside the external ear canal. Otoscopes come with an assortment of little funnels with various-size ends for various-size ear canals. Use the largest size funnel which will fit comfortably into the canal you are examining. If the funnel size is too small, it is very difficult to see anything at all.

5. Under direct observation, still pulling the ear flap backward, slowly insert the otoscope down the ear canal as far as it will comfortably and easily go, *as long as you see nothing in the path ahead.* It is important to look through the otoscope as you insert it because there may be some wax there or a foreign body such as a stone or a bean in the ear. By inserting the otoscope without watching, you could actually push this further into the ear canal and do serious damage. It cannot be stressed too strongly that if you use an otoscope, you must watch where you are going.

6. The normal ear canal is a light tan color with just a blush of pink in it. You may also see a very dark, reddish brown material about the

consistency and color of very thick automobile grease. This is ear wax and should be no cause for concern. Sometimes the wax only partially obstructs the canal and you can complete your examination by looking past it. You may find, however, that your view of the external auditory canal and the eardrum is entirely blocked by wax. If this is the case, you will have to remove it before you can complete your observations.

Ear wax is easily removed by first softening the wax for several days with a drugstore preparation called Debrox, as described below. Before you go ahead with this procedure, however, there is one very important precaution regarding the use of Debrox and the washing procedure which it involves. Sometimes as a result of a previous accident or infection, the eardrum has been ruptured, resulting in a permanent hole in the drum. You can see such a hole in the eardrum with your otoscope if wax does not obscure it. If you know or suspect that you have a hole in your eardrum, you should not use Debrox nor should you squirt water into your ear. Water can do permanent damage to the middle ear, so the ear-washing procedure described below should not be carried out if there is a hole in the eardrum.

Removing Ear Wax

1. Administer several drops of Debrox in the ear twice a day for two or three days.

2. You will find that the wax becomes so soft that it almost runs out. The ear can now be cleaned using an ear-cleaning syringe: a simple rubber squeeze bulb is quite adequate for this purpose. Before you proceed to rinse the ear out, look into it with your otoscope and make certain that the wax is soft and runny. If it still looks quite hard, give the Debrox another day or two to work.

3. To wash out the ear, fill the syringe with warm water and *gently* squirt the water into the ear canal. Place the pointed tip of the ear syringe very loosely into the canal. You must not completely block the canal with the tip of the syringe or the water you are squirting in will have no place to go. You can do permanent harm to your ear by plugging the canal tightly with the tip of a rubber ear syringe and then squeezing hard.

4. With the tip of the syringe loosely inserted, the water will come running right back out, mixed with chunks of softened ear wax.

Ear wax is not the only material which may be found in the external ear canal. Small foreign objects often find their way into the ear, especially in young children. Unless the foreign object you find is a piece of cotton which you can easily grab with a tweezers, do not attempt to remove it yourself. Specially designed tweezers are generally required for hard objects and attempts to remove a foreign object yourself will more often lead to accidentally pushing it further in than actually retrieving it. It is very difficult to grasp a foreign object in the ear canal using conventional tweezers. Go to your doctor and have it done for you.

One other condition which you might conceivably find is a wet, greenish substance indicating an infection of the external ear canal. This is invariably accompanied by some degree of discomfort. An infection of the external ear canal should be promptly treated with the appropriate antibiotic ear drops. Thus if your initial inspection reveals a greenish, wet, messy-looking ear canal, you should visit your doctor without delay.

Inspecting the Eardrum

Once you have made certain that there is no ear wax, no foreign body and no infection present in the external ear canal, you should be able to observe the eardrum using your otoscope.

1. Following the previous instructions regarding the use of an otoscope (reread the method for inspecting the external ear canal in "Using an Otoscope"), straighten the ear canal by pulling the external ear flap firmly backward and insert the otoscope down the ear canal as far as it will easily and comfortably go. Remember: Always look into the otoscope as you perform your inspection to make absolutely certain that you have a clear and unobstructed path.

2. If you have straightened the canal correctly, you should now be able to identify the eardrum. The eardrum, as you will recall, is a cone-shaped membrane stretched across the inner end of the external auditory canal. A common error in ear examinations is to mistake the canal wall for the drum. The walls of the external auditory canal and the eardrum are normally a dull, slightly pinkish tan. The eardrum, however, is a bit shiny compared to the canal wall and should reflect light back to you.

3. Under direct observation, move your otoscope around a bit both up and down and from side to side until you get a clear view of the drum. There is a small protrusion at one point where the middle ear bones are attached on the inside. This gives the eardrum the appearance of the top of a slightly rounded tent with the tent pole sticking up at you just a little.

4. Study the appearance of the eardrum carefully. An infection of the

middle ear can affect the appearance of the eardrum in several ways. The mildest effect is simply a slight graying of color and a loss of the normal light reflection. Another form of middle ear infection is indicated by a bluish eardrum. If an infection of the middle ear continues unchecked, the eardrum will become pink and eventually quite bright red. If an advanced middle ear infection is present and the Eustachian tube is blocked, the eardrum may bulge considerably. A bulging, inflamed-looking eardrum indicates a severe infection of the middle ear. It will also be quite painful. If this goes unattended, the eardrum may rupture, resulting in substantial and sometimes permanent hearing loss. Should your examination reveal a bulging, red drum, or an eardrum with a gray or bluish cast, you should seek medical attention immediately.

After a middle ear infection has been treated, the eardrum gradually returns to its normal, slightly rounded shape and recovers its slightly shiny surface. Sometimes a dark redness lingers around the edges of the drum as the infection clears up.

Even without an otoscope, it is possible to learn quite a bit about the ear simply by observing any discharge which comes out of the auditory canal. The wet, greenish substance which is characteristic of an external ear canal infection usually comes running out at some point. With such infections the ear canal always feels painful or at least strange, and there is always some hearing loss on the affected side.

Ear wax occasionally becomes fluid enough to run out of the ear, particularly at night if you sleep with your ear pressed against the pillow. The insulating qualities of the pillow warm up that side of your head just a bit, causing the wax to soften and run out of the ear. You may notice this on your pillow in the morning as a dry, crusted material and mistake it for blood. If you are unable to distinguish between ear wax and dried blood, and you have reason to believe that your ear has bled, you should test the substance for traces of blood using the test described below.

Bleeding from the Ear.   Blood coming from the ear canal is a serious finding. It is never normal. There are a few very ordinary, unimportant reasons for ear bleeding such as pimples at the entrance to the canal, but in general the symptom is likely to be a serious one and should not be ignored. If you suspect that blood has come from your ear canal, you can quickly confirm your suspicions—or lay them to rest—using the following test.

Testing for Bleeding from the Ear

You can test unknown substances from the ear canal for blood with the same Hematest® kit you use to test for blood in the stools (refer to the chapter on the digestive process). The Hematest® kit will detect traces of blood—if any are present—in a sample of material from the ear canal. You should be able to purchase these kits in any well-stocked pharmacy, particularly one attached to a medical center or a professional building.

1. The Hematest® kit consists of a bottle of reagent tablets and special filter paper. Place a sample of the crusty dried material on the impregnated test paper.
2. Following the instructions that come with the kit, place a reagent tablet in the center of the specimen on the filter paper.
3. Place one drop of water on the tablet and allow 5 to 10 seconds for the water to penetrate the tablet. Then add a second drop so that the water runs down the side of the tablet onto the specimen and filter paper. Gently tap the side of the tablet once or twice to knock off water droplets from the top of the tablet.
4. Wait 2 minutes and observe the filter paper for a color change indicating the presence of blood. Blood will give a very strong, positive blue reaction. Ear wax will give practically no color at all except for perhaps a little spreading of the brown tinge. A positive reaction from this test indicates bleeding from the ear canal, and you should consult your doctor without delay.

Hearing and Hearing Loss.   Since the primary function of the ear is to hear, hearing testing is the best criterion of whether or not the ear is working properly. (A secondary function, balance, is dealt with in the chapter on the nervous system.)

Human hearing is measured according to two scales. One scale tests your range of pitch—that is, the lowest and the highest tones which you can hear. This is measured in terms of cycles per second. Normal conversation registers about 1000 cycles; a 6000-cycle tone sounds like a very high squeak. Average human hearing ranges from a low of 20 to a high of 20,000 cycles per second. High-frequency hearing decreases with age, down to about 8000 cycles per second for a fifty-year-old individual, and 4000 for an eighty-year-old. Rock-group musicians and their audiences whose ears have been assaulted by very loud music over a long period of time are especially vulnerable to high-frequency hearing loss.

A second scale—the decibel scale—measures human hearing in

terms of intensity, or loudness. A whisper from four feet away measures about 20 decibels, and a normal conversation registers about 60 decibels.

Hearing is generally tested using an audiometer—a rather sophisticated piece of electronic equipment that measures both intensity of sound (loudness) and frequency (pitch). You cannot duplicate audiometer testing in your home, of course. However, it should be apparent from the preceding discussion that we ordinarily use only a small part of our total hearing range, and that is the voice range. We are not commonly called upon to discern very high, very low, or very soft sounds.

There are a number of observations you can make which may lead you to suspect that you or someone else in the family is suffering from a hearing deficiency:

• Seeming inattention when someone speaks
• Continually asking what? or huh?
• Difficulty hearing on the telephone
• Learning difficulties in school
• Difficulty in learning to speak
• A habit of speaking considerably louder than seems necessary

Naturally, all of these habits may have other causes besides hearing loss, but any one of them should prompt you to consider a hearing test to be sure everything is all right. There are several ways you can test your hearing at home to see if more extensive, professional testing is warranted.

Testing for Hearing Loss
Method 1. You will need a ticking watch and a tape measure for this test. An easy method to quickly screen for hearing loss is to see how far away a ticking watch can be heard by a person known to have good hearing. Compare this with the farthest distance the *same* watch can be heard by the person being tested. Start at a distance where you are sure the watch is too far away to be heard and gradually bring it closer.

Method 2. You will need two telephone extensions in different rooms and a cassette recorder for this test:
a. Record a series of names and numbers on a tape recorder. Speak quietly, slowly, and distinctly, allowing enough time between items for a listener to write down the name or number. Keep your voice level; do not vary the volume.
b. Call the telephone company repair service and ask how you can dial your own number to talk from one extension to another.

c. After dialing your extension phone, play the recording at low volume into one phone while the test subject listens on the other phone. Move the recorder further away from the phone as each name or number is recited.

d. The subject being tested writes down what he or she can hear.

e. Compare the subject's ability to hear with that of someone known to have good hearing who takes the same test.

Method 3.

a. With the subject seated across the room from a radio, record player, or tape player, play a voice recording or tune in a news broadcast.

b. Start with the volume turned down to where no sound can be heard. Turn the volume up very slowly until the subject can repeat what is being said. You must turn the volume knob very slowly because the sound comes up very quickly.

c. Compare the subject's voice range hearing with that of a person known to have good hearing.

There are also checks for hearing loss that can be done with a tuning fork. A tuning fork rated at 256 cycles per second is commonly used. The cost of such an instrument is about $10 to $15 at a medical supply store, or you may find one you can borrow at a local high-school physics laboratory.

Testing Hearing Using a Tuning Fork

Method 1.

a. Strike the tuning fork to make it vibrate.

b. Place the end of the stem of the fork against the skull behind the ear.

c. Ask the subject being tested to report when the sound can no longer be heard.

d. At this point, immediately bring the prongs of the fork to the subject's ear opening. If hearing is normal, a faint sound will again be heard by the subject.

Method 2.

a. Strike the tuning fork to make it vibrate.

b. Place the end of the stem on top of the subject's head at about the center.

c. If the sound is louder in one ear than in the other, it indicates some loss of hearing. (To understand this effect better, try it yourself and plug one ear at a time with your finger. The sound becomes dramatically loud in the unplugged ear.)

THE NOSE

Our modern, deodorized society pays scant homage to the lowly nose. More reviled than revered, the hapless proboscis has taken a back seat to the eyes and ears ever since man started walking upright with his nose in the air instead of on the ground. Yet it little deserves its status as a poor cousin to the other senses. The average nose identifies about four thousand different smells, and the trained nose of a perfumer can distinguish up to ten thousand different scents. And if you were suddenly deprived of your vision and hearing, your nose would really come into its own, identifying people, houses, and even rooms by the sense of smell alone.

What you think of as your nose is actually two noses, one on either side of the septum—that partition of bone and cartilage which runs down the middle of the nasal cavity.

One of the primary functions of the nose is to clean and condition the air we breathe before it reaches the delicate tissues in the lungs. Long, coarse hairs just inside each nostril, and the mucous membranes—spongy red tissue lining the nasal cavity—filter out dust and other contaminants and help warm and humidify cold, dry air. This latter function is assisted greatly by the nasal turbinates. These are three little chips of bone, the biggest about an inch long, which protrude from the upper septum in each nostril. The nasal turbinates are also covered by mucous membrane. When you breathe in cold air, this tissue swells with blood, providing a greater surface area for warming the frigid air.

The other function of the nose, of course, is smell. The olfactory area of your nose is contained in a surprisingly small patch of tissue about the size of a postage stamp, yellow-brown in color, located in the roof of each nostril.

Finally, the nasal chamber also includes the eight sinus cavities. These are hollow pockets in the surrounding bone lined with the same mucous membrane found in the nasal passages. While the sinus cavities serve to lighten the skull (solid bone would add considerably to the weight of the skull) and add resonance to our voice, they are often troublesome. The sinuses communicate with the rest of the nasal cavity via narrow channels that are easily infected. When this happens, the opening into the main chamber becomes swollen and closes, and pressure builds up within the sinus cavity, causing considerable pain and discomfort. This inflammation of the mucous membrane lining these air spaces is called sinusitis. Since the sinuses are enclosed by bone, you will not be able to observe them in your examination of the nose.

Observing the External Nose

An external examination of the nose involves a critical look at its shape, color, and configuration.

The nose is normally bilaterally symmetric—that is, one side should look much like the other—and the midline, or bridge, should be straight. If the midline of the nose is shifted markedly to one side, this is an indication of an abnormality, usually the result of a trauma, or accident.

A bulbous, red nose is definitely abnormal but, contrary to popular belief, it is not necessarily an indication of alcoholism. A condition called acne rosacea, caused by excessive flushing of the blood vessels in the nose and cheek, also causes a red nose, and so do certain vitamin deficiencies and infections.

A general enlargement of the tissues of the nose can also occur. There are several types of disorders which can cause this, most of which are fairly rare.

If your nose has taken on a red, bulbous appearance or seems larger than normal, you should bring these findings to the attention of your doctor.

An internal examination of the nose can be carried out using either a penlight or a nasal speculum. If you have purchased an otoscope, you probably already have a nasal speculum. This is the largest of the little funnels which come with the otoscope. Somewhat shorter and fatter than the rest, it is specially designed for looking into the nose. If you don't have one of these, you can do almost as well by looking into the nose with just a penlight.

Examining the Inside of the Nose

1. Press the tip of the nose inward to widen the openings and peer upward into the nasal cavity. If you are using a nasal speculum, you must take the same care you took when inspecting the ear. That means never insert the instrument up the nostril without looking where you are going. Check to make sure that there are no foreign objects that could be pushed further into the nasal cavity by your speculum. As with the ear, if a foreign object is lodged fairly far into the nose, special instruments are required to retrieve it and this should not be attempted at home.

2. Examine the mucous membrane which lines the inside of the nose. This is normally pinkish in color and is covered with a number of fine hairs. When you come down with a cold, this lining becomes swollen and reddened. The nose feels stuffy and a watery discharge is present. As the cold wears on, this discharge becomes somewhat

thickened and yellow. During an allergic nasal reaction such as hay fever, the mucous membrane also becomes swollen. In this case, however, the swollen membrane is rather pale in color and the discharge, while profuse, is quite watery.

3. Inspect the central nasal septum. This is the wall between the two nostrils. The septum should be straight and smooth, its mucous membrane pinkish. A hole in the septum is not normal. Should you discover a perforation, you should seek medical advice promptly.

4. Locate the nasal turbinates. Higher up in the nasal cavity, up either side of the septum, are three small, shelflike protrusions. These are the nasal turbinates and they, too, are covered with the same mucous membrane that lines the rest of the cavity. You may not be able to see the turbinates without a nasal speculum.

5. Look for polyps. These are boggy, swollen, sac-like masses that can block air passages and sinus channels. They resemble little mushrooms and may be quite small or as large as a grape. Polyps are often found in conjunction with allergies. These should be reported to a physician.

Your examination of the nose should conclude with a test of your ability to perceive different odors. Our sense of smell is controlled by the olfactory nerve, which is the first cranial nerve. A test of first cranial nerve function can be found in the chapter titled "Testing the Nervous System."

THE MOUTH

Just about everyone has trouble with his or her teeth and gums at some point. Luckily, the mouth is a fitting subject for self-examination simply because it is so conveniently situated and because abnormalities are so readily apparent once you know what you're looking for. You can diagnose a number of abnormal conditions and get a good look inside this vital cavity with the aid of a few simple tools. You will need a penlight, a wooden tongue blade, and a dental mirror. You can purchase an inexpensive plastic dental mirror and tongue blades at most drugstores. The handle of a teaspoon may be used in place of a tongue blade.

The Tongue.   A good place to start your inspection of the mouth is with the tongue. The tongue is a complex assortment of muscles and nerves enclosed in mucous membrane. The mucous membrane covering is studded with taste buds on both the top and bottom surfaces.

These taste buds transmit sour, bitter, sweet, and salty taste sensations to the brain via special nerves. You can test your sense of taste by checking this aspect of seventh and ninth cranial nerve function with the tests found in the chapter titled "Testing the Nervous System." Another cranial nerve, the twelfth, controls the muscles of the tongue; this too is tested with the nervous system. In addition to detecting taste sensations, the tongue is an invaluable aid in preparing food for the digestive process and in the formation of speech sounds.

Inspecting the Tongue

You can get the best view of your tongue by grasping the tip with a small, 4 × 4-inch piece of clean cloth and gently pulling it into view in front of your bathroom mirror. Hint: Rub warm water over the mirror to prevent it from fogging up when you breathe on it.

1. Inspect the size, shape, and color of your tongue. The surface of the tongue should be pink and somewhat rough. Observe the coating on top of the tongue. It is normally a whitish-gray color that may be more noticeable on some days than others. Smokers typically have a heavier coating on their tongues, particularly in the morning after they get up. A greenish-white fungus sometimes appears on the surface of the tongue, and if you have been taking antibiotics, your tongue may have a black coating. But neither these nor most other discolorations of a normally rough tongue are of serious consequence. A smooth, beefy-red tongue, however, is abnormal and occurs in several diseases.

The shape of the tongue may vary from one person to another; some tongues are flat and pointed while others are fuller and more rounded.

If you have ever been fitted for dentures after going without teeth for some time, your tongue probably felt too big for your mouth. That's because your tongue grew a bit to take up the extra space left by the missing teeth. When these are replaced, the tongue eventually shrinks to a more appropriate size for your mouth area. If your tongue feels too big for your mouth or seems to have shrunk, and you have not recently either lost or acquired your teeth, you should bring this to the attention of your dentist.

2. Identify the taste buds. Blot your tongue dry with a paper towel and observe it closely using your penlight. You should be able to see the taste buds. They look a bit like bunches of tiny strings or soft, miniature brushes. As mentioned above, the sensation of taste is controlled by cranial nerves, which are tested in the chapter "Testing the Nervous System."

3. Look for sores. Observe all surfaces of the tongue for lumps, open

sores, ulcers, swellings, pain, or tenderness. None of these conditions are normal and any that persist for longer than a week should receive medical attention.

Salivary Glands.   Your mouth also contains a vital gland that is often overlooked and unappreciated and that is the salivary gland. There are three of them, actually, one in each cheek and one under the tongue. The saliva produced by these glands lubricates your food, aids in swallowing food and digesting it, and plays a role in fighting tooth decay by neutralizing acid in the mouth. You should be able to locate your salivary glands and observe them in action.

Checking the Salivary Ducts

Holding your cheek out a bit with your fingers, run your tongue blade along the inside of your cheek. This will tend to exaggerate any bumps. You should notice a little pimplelike bump in the middle of the cheek, opposite the upper last two teeth. This is the outlet of the salivary duct, from which saliva is introduced into the mouth. You will find one on each cheek. A third duct is located under the tongue, directly behind the lower front teeth.

You can observe the function of the salivary ducts with this simple test. Do not eat, drink, or chew gum for a few hours. This lulls the salivary glands into a resting state. Then chew on a sugared slice of lemon for about five seconds or so. Now look at the salivary gland outlets again and you should be able to see saliva pouring from the ducts.

Check all three ducts. The outlets do occasionally get plugged up. In such cases the saliva backs up in the duct, the gland swells, and becomes very painful. If this happens, you should see your doctor at once.

Inspecting Your Teeth.   A thorough inspection of your teeth can reveal a variety of potentially troublesome conditions including cavities, unnatural gaps, the presence of plaque, improper bite, tooth sensitivity, stains, and nerve damage.

Before beginning your inspection, brush your teeth and then rinse thoroughly with lukewarm water. Run warm water over your dental mirror to keep it from fogging up during your examination.

Checking for Cavities

Cavities are most commonly found in three areas: between the teeth, at the gum line, and in the grooves on the tops of the teeth. A cavity is indicated by a small hole, usually stained by a blackish color. (The hole on the outside, by the way, is very much smaller than the hole being made on the inside.)

Examine each tooth in your mouth carefully and methodically for evidence of decay. You may prefer to work with a partner and inspect each other's teeth. In order to view all surfaces of your teeth, you will have to use your penlight in coordination with your dental mirror. To do this, hold your dental mirror behind the tooth surface which you wish to observe, shine the penlight *into the mirror* and let it reflect its light onto the tooth. In this way, the mirror serves to bend the light directly onto a hidden surface. Use your mirror to help keep your tongue out of the way. All of this takes some coordination, but you should be able to master the technique with a bit of practice.

Be sure not to miss any tooth surface in your examination. If you find a suspicious spot, make a note of it and report to your dentist.

The normal complement of adult teeth is thirty-two. This includes your four wisdom teeth which you may have had pulled, or which may be hidden in the gum. Starting with the tooth furthest back in your upper right jaw, count your teeth. You will need to use your dental mirror to do this; don't go by touch alone. If you have fewer than twenty-eight teeth, you should carefully examine the gaps where teeth are missing.

Examining Unnatural Gaps

Where a tooth (or teeth) is missing, check the corresponding tooth in the other jaw to see if it is growing into the void left by the missing tooth. To do this, close your jaws and then separate your lips with your fingers; look at the tooth opposite the empty space to see if it extends down (or up) further than the teeth on either side of it. If you find this to be so, you should bring it to the attention of your dentist without delay. If any of your teeth have begun to move or grow into a space where a tooth is missing, this too is a serious finding that requires professional attention.

Plaque is a sticky, almost invisible film composed of bacteria, saliva, and food debris that clings to tooth surfaces, eventually causing tooth decay and gum disease. You can check your teeth for evidence of plaque by using disclosing tablets. These tablets, available at most pharmacies, contain a harmless dye which will turn plaque bright red so you can locate and remove it more effectively. Do not be concerned

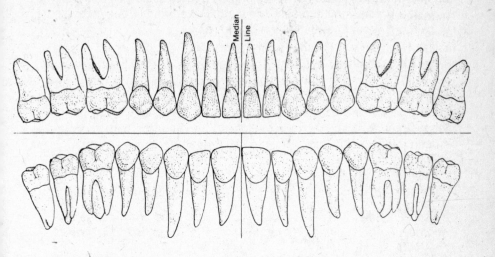

about the tablet staining the inside of your mouth; the color will disappear within a few hours.

Testing for Plaque
After cleaning your teeth, chew a disclosing tablet well, let it dissolve in your saliva, and swish it around in your mouth; then empty your mouth. Examine your mouth using your penlight and dental mirror as described earlier so that you can observe both the inner and outer surfaces of your teeth. The red-stained areas represent deposits of plaque that can be removed with more thorough brushing and flossing.

An improper bite, called malocclusion, is one in which the teeth do not come together uniformly and evenly. Many of us have some degree of malocclusion; a common form is jaw-to-jaw mismatch in which either the upper or the lower jaw protrudes. Malocclusion can also result from crooked teeth and from high fillings. A high filling, as the name implies, is slightly higher than the teeth on either side. Thus when you bite, you will be hitting first on this spot.

Checking for High Spots on Silver Fillings
You can check for high spots that can result in malocclusion by taking your dental mirror and penlight and looking for a shiny spot on an

otherwise dull silver filling. Should you find such a spot, or if when you bite down without food in your mouth you seem to be hitting first on just one side of your mouth, or just one tooth or the filling of one tooth, you should bring this to the attention of your dentist.

Healthy teeth should not be particularly sensitive to pressure or hot or cold sensations. If you have a tooth which you suspect is unsound, test it for unusual sensitivity.

Testing for Tooth Sensitivity

If you have reason to believe that a particular tooth is unsound, gently tap its upper surface with a spoon handle. If it hurts or is even moderately sensitive, there is probably something wrong with the root or inner pulp of the tooth. A normal tooth does not hurt when you tap it with a spoon handle. If there is a question in your mind concerning the response of a particular tooth, tap the same tooth on the other side of the jaw for comparison.

Next, swish some hot water and then cold water around in your mouth. Neither of these should cause you any undue discomfort. Once in a while your teeth may react to extreme temperatures, but persistent temperature sensitivity in one or more teeth is not normal and should be brought to the attention of your dentist.

Stains on the teeth can be yellow, orange, brown, red, and even green. Most of them are harmless (as long as they are not hiding evidence of decay) and can be removed with a professional cleaning. You should be concerned, however, about dark stains in a tooth that was recently white and healthy-looking, because this may indicate damage to the nerve root.

Diagnosing Nerve Damage in a Tooth

A discoloration in just one tooth or in two adjacent teeth that were white and healthy-looking a short time ago should be viewed with suspicion, particularly if you recently received a blow to the mouth. (Note: Children commonly get struck in the mouth in the course of play and may not recall the incident several days later.) A blow to the mouth does not have to be powerful to kill the nerve in a tooth, just well placed.

If the nerve root is damaged, the tooth begins to die, changing color in the process. This color change can range from gray to yellow to brown or black. If you notice this kind of localized discoloration in a recently healthy tooth, you should treat it as a dental emergency.

An inspection of your teeth is not complete without a close examination of your gums. Normal, healthy gums have five characteristics: (1) They are firm and fit snugly around each tooth. (2) They are pinkish in color or even whitish-pink. An exception to this is dark-skinned people, particularly blacks, whose gums are darker in color. (3) Gum tissue forms a V between the teeth. (4) Gums have little dotlike indentations, called stippling, especially in the areas closest to the teeth. (5) Gum tissue forms tiny "collars" around the base of each tooth. To identify these last two characteristics, you will need to blot dry a section of gum tissue and observe it closely using your penlight.

Gum disease can take many forms and is an insidious process which leads, if unchecked, to substantial tooth loss. You can spot gum disease at an early stage, when it is still treatable, by performing the following inspection at frequent intervals.

Checking for Signs of Gum Disease

Keeping in mind how normal, healthy gums look, examine your gums for the five characteristics described above. Use your dental mirror and penlight to examine hard-to-see areas of gum tissue. As you perform your inspection, check for these telltale signs of gum disease.

1. Bleeding gums. Healthy gums do not bleed. If your gums bleed during brushing or while eating, they are not normal. If you are not sure if your gums bleed or not, gently run a length of dental floss between two teeth and against the area of gum in question. If this procedure causes the gum to bleed, this is an abnormal finding that probably indicates some degree of gum disease.

2. Pus in gums. A white, puslike substance exuding from the tip of the gums is abnormal. If the tip of the gum between the teeth looks white and pus-filled, put your finger on the gum and press inward and upward. Traces of pus or blood as a result of this procedure are abnormal.

3. Receding gums. The gums should appear to be attached to the enamel, or white part, of the tooth. If the gum appears to be receding from the tooth, thus exposing more of the tooth and even the root to view, this should be brought to the attention of your dentist without delay.

4. Swollen, puffy, red gums. Gums that are angry or inflamed-looking are unhealthy. Check closely around the base of each tooth for this abnormal reddening.

5. Painful, burning gums. Gums that are tender to the touch and have a stinging, burning sensation are probably diseased.

Gum disease is also likely to be accompanied by bad breath and, in advanced cases, a slight fever as well. Never underestimate the role of a healthy mouth in your general well-being. It is a mistake to assume that a toothache or gum disease is of minor consequence. Like any threat to your system, they draw upon the body's resources to mobilize an attack against the invading infection; this is a debilitating process that saps your vitality. If the infection continues unchecked, your teeth will be only the first casualty in what can be a long, miserable war.

THE THROAT

Examining the throat requires working with a partner. The landmarks of the throat can be identified rather easily using a penlight and a tongue depressor. (The handle of a spoon may be substituted for a wooden tongue blade.)

Ask your partner to open his or her mouth wide and relax the tongue. In many people you will be able to see the throat clearly without the aid of a tongue depressor. If you have trouble seeing past the tongue, place the tongue blade or spoon handle on the surface of the tongue about two-thirds of the way back and press down gently. You must be gentle but firm when doing this, and position the tongue blade carefully. If it is placed too far back on the tongue, you are likely to gag your subject and not see anything. If your tongue blade is too far forward, you will not be able to press down enough of the tongue to improve your view of the throat.

Shine your flashlight into the mouth. (If you purchased an otoscope for examining the ear, check to see if your otoscope head converts into a throat illuminator.) With the tongue out of the way, you should be able to see the throat clearly. The wall at the very rear of the mouth

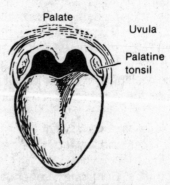

The Palatine Tonsils

belongs to a tube called the pharynx which connects the nasal cavity with the oral cavity and continues on down to the esophagus and, eventually, the stomach. One obvious landmark here is a little tongue of tissue that hangs down from the roof of the mouth to the center of the throat. This is not, as many people mistakenly believe, a tonsil. This is the uvula, and every time you swallow it acts as a flap, closing off the passage to the nasal cavity and thereby insuring that your meal goes down the pharynx instead of up your nose. Your tonsils are located on either side of the uvula, behind little curtains of tissue. These little curtains on each side of the rear wall of the mouth are called the tonsilar pillars. The tonsils protrude out a bit from behind the tonsilar pillars, one on either side.

Examining the Tonsils

Using your flashlight and tongue blade in the procedure described above, locate the tonsils and the tonsilar pillars.

Like the membranes inside the nose and mouth, the tonsilar pillars and the tonsils should be uniformly pinkish in color. The tonsils are normally about the size of a cherry, and the surface is covered with a series of irregular, barely visible grooves. Healthy tonsils are often almost completely hidden behind the tonsilar pillars.

When the throat becomes infected, the tonsils enlarge dramatically, particularly in children, and all the tissues of the throat become red and inflamed. Infected tonsils may also show patches of white material in the normal cracks and grooves on the surface. White patches on the tonsils are characteristic of streptococcal infections, known as strep throat, and are therefore an important finding. Anyone who has a fever, a sore throat, swollen lymph nodes at the angle of the jaw and along the front of the neck (more about lymph node enlargement later), and enlarged tonsils with patches of white should see his or her doctor promptly.

If left untreated, a streptococcal infection can lead to far more serious problems than a sore throat. Scarlet fever, for one, is actually a generalized streptococcal infection which has spread through the whole body. One of the more serious types of valvular heart disease is caused by a streptococcal infection of the heart following a strep throat. Uncontrolled, this can do extensive damage which will eventually require open-heart surgery. The kidneys, too, are a potential target for the streptococcal bacteria. It is primarily with the hope of avoiding these life-threatening aftereffects that physicians are so anxious to treat streptococcal infections. It is an easy disease to treat, as virtually all strains of the bacteria are presently sensitive to penicillin. If you suspect you have strep throat, you should immediately consult a doctor.

THE NECK

While the head is surely our crowning glory, the neck on which it sits is more than just an elegant pedestal. Along with the bony spinal column and a system of muscles which, together, allow us to hold the head at innumerable angles, the neck also contains many of the lymph nodes which help combat infections, the thyroid gland which fine-tunes our body's throttle, so to speak, and the major arteries which supply blood to the brain. Normally, our neck presents a very unremarkable exterior. It can, however, be a revealing indicator of a number of disease states.

The Lymph Nodes.   Enlarged lymph nodes are a sure sign that the body is fighting off an infection of some kind. The lymph nodes are little nodules of tissue which function as filters for our body fluids. Most of the time these nodes are too small to be seen or felt. But when the body has been invaded by infection, the lymph nodes trap bacteria, viruses, and other debris traveling through the bloodstream. As a node accumulates more and more material, it enlarges and you can feel it quite readily.

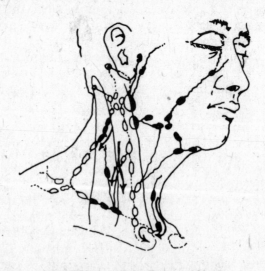

Lymph Nodes of the Face and Neck

The body has a large number of lymph nodes located in the neck, in the armpits, behind and above the elbows, in the area of the groin, and in the hollow of each collarbone. Different lymph nodes drain different parts of the body. Knowing which nodes filter which areas can help you to identify the probable source of an infection.

There are a number of lymph nodes located in the region of the head and neck, as indicated in the following drawing. These nodes may become enlarged singly or in groups.

Examining the Lymph Nodes in the Neck

With your fingers together, use the fleshy pads of the fingers to feel for lymph nodes along the entire course of the neck. Try to relax your neck muscles while you do this. Make sure your examination extends around to the back of the neck, up under the chin, and at the angle of the jaw as well.

A swollen lymph node may feel soft or hard, and may or may not be painful when you press on it. But usually a node that has enlarged due to a simple infection feels soft and is painful when you poke at it.

Under normal circumstances, you will not find any lumps at all. A number of common and not-so-common infections, however, can cause the lymph nodes to enlarge.

You are most likely to find swollen lymph nodes under the jaw. These nodes commonly swell as a reaction to a toothache, sores in the mouth, or a viral respiratory infection such as the flu. Swollen nodes behind the ears suggest German measles or an ear infection, whereas enlarged nodes in front of the ears point to some problem in the area of the face and eyes. Finally, all the lymph nodes in your body may be swollen in response to a generalized infection such as mononucleosis.

While these general rules usually prove to be an accurate guide to the source of an infection, it is not unheard of for a lymph node to respond to an infection in some other node's territory. If the source of an infection is not obvious, or if any swollen node does not subside within a week's time, you should see your doctor.

The Thyroid Gland.   The thyroid gland, located just below your Adam's apple, should also be examined. The thyroid is a butterfly-shaped gland situated over the trachea, or windpipe, with one "wing" on either side. Its main function is to control metabolism—that is, the rate at which our cells burn food to convert into energy. It does this by producing tiny amounts of hormones which are released into the bloodstream upon instructions from the master endocrine gland, the pituitary, which is located at the base of the brain.

Locating the Thyroid Gland

Except in very thin people, it is difficult to actually feel a normal thyroid gland. It is, however, the only gland in the neck that moves when you swallow. Thus if you locate your Adam's apple and press your fingers lightly but firmly over the area immediately below, you should be able to feel the thyroid gland move beneath your fingers as you drink a glass of water.

The thyroid gland may become enlarged, in which case it is known as a goiter. Men may first notice the presence of a goiter when they have difficulty buttoning a shirt collar. Women may first notice it as a puffiness in the front of the neck. Such a swelling may feel hard or soft, smooth or lumpy, and may vary in size from barely visible to grossly distended. Any thyroid gland which you can locate with your eyes alone, without the aid of the swallow test, is abnormally enlarged and should be examined by your doctor.

The thyroid gland may become either underactive or overactive in its hormone production, and this can happen without any telltale changes in size.

A thyroid hormone deficiency, called hypothyroidism, is indicated by a combination of symptoms. These include an increase in the amount of sleep you require every day, a moderate weight gain that is not associated with increased hunger, or even an increased food intake, dry skin, brittle, coarse hair, and a chronic tired and sluggish feeling. If this picture seems to fit you, the following test is useful in helping decide if your problem is due to a thyroid hormone deficiency.

Testing for an Underactive Thyroid

This test involves the knee-jerk reflex which is also described in the chapter on the nervous system. Here, however, you will be observing not so much the knee jerk itself as the relaxation stage of the reflex when the lower leg returns to its normal position. The knee-jerk test is best carried out with some help from an assistant.

1. Sit on a table so that your legs swing freely from the knee joint, with your knees bared.
2. Locate your kneecap with your fingers. This is the rounded bone which sits right over the knee.
3. Next, locate a bony prominence an inch or so below the kneecap.

This is the top end of the large bone in your lower leg. In the very front part of your leg you will feel a fairly stiff cord running in this short space between the bottom of the kneecap and the top of the leg bone. You should actually be able to put your thumb and index finger on either side of this cord. You are now holding the tendon you are about to test. Mark this point with an X using a felt-tip pen.

4. With your legs totally relaxed, ask your assistant to briskly tap each knee with a rubber reflex hammer at the point you have marked. It is very important to relax or the test will not work properly. Remember, it is a *tap* you deliver, not a blow.

5. In most people, if the test is done correctly, the lower leg will immediately give a little jerk. Normally, the lower leg will relax promptly. When thyroid hormone production is deficient, however, the leg sinks slowly back to its former position. This sluggish relaxation phase of the deep tendon reflex is characteristic of an underactive thyroid.

The thyroid can become overactive as well as underactive in its production of the hormone governing our metabolism. An overactive thyroid condition is called *hyper*thyroidism and it, too, is characterized by a combination of symptoms.

People suffering from hyperthyroidism almost always lose weight, even when they increase their food intake, their skin feels moist, they perspire excessively, their heart rate is rapid, they feel nervous and jittery, and they often exhibit exophthalmia. In common terms, this is called "pop eyes" and it actually looks as if the eyes are slowly bulging out of their sockets. The first sign of this is just a slightly wide-eyed look. Normally the upper eyelid rests over part of the iris, which is the colored part of the eye. But as the eye bulges out, the lid is raised higher and higher and more and more of the upper part of the iris is exposed.

A good test for an overactive thyroid is the tremor test.

Testing for an Overactive Thyroid

Hold one hand out in front of you with the back side up. Stretch all the fingers out as far as they will go. Now lay an ordinary sheet of paper on the back of your hand. Watch the edges of this paper carefully. In a few people the edges will remain absolutely still. In most, the edges will wiggle a little. If you have an overactive thyroid, however, the edges of the paper will vibrate quite violently. No matter how still you try to hold your hand, the paper will still dance around.

While people may develop hand tremors for many reasons, a significant tremor in combination with a loss of weight, slightly bulging eyes, and a feeling of nervousness is very suggestive of hyperthyroidism, and a physician should be consulted.

The Carotid Arteries.   We've all seen it done in countless spy movies—the secret agent steps up to his victim and places his fingers over a strategic spot on the neck, whereupon the victim drops neatly to the ground. This mysterious little maneuver involves one of the two carotid arteries in the neck which carry blood to the brain. And while the old fingers-on-the-neck stunt is more a *tour de force* than a lethal weapon, the carotid arteries are indeed both vital and vulnerable.

Arteries carry blood from the heart to all parts of the body. The two carotid arteries start at the heart and pass through the neck on their way to the brain. One artery supplies one side of the brain and the other artery provides blood for the other half. Any interruption or slackening of the supply of blood to the brain can have tragic consequences.

Like any other arteries, the carotid arteries can become narrowed or blocked, leading to a stroke. You can make a basic evaluation of these two vital arteries yourself with a few simple observations and the use of your stethoscope.

Examining the Carotid Arteries

1. The first step in your evaluation of the carotid arteries consists of visual observation. The two carotid arteries enter the neck behind the two bony prominences at the base of the neck commonly known as the collarbones. Carefully observe this area of the neck. Except during vigorous physical exertion or extreme emotional distress, you should not be able to detect with your eyes the pulsation of the carotid arteries. These arteries may throb visibly, however, in aged people and in those suffering from high blood pressure, hyperthyroidism, and anemia. If you are able to see the pulsation of the carotid arteries in your neck, you should bring this finding to the attention of your doctor.

2. Now locate the pulse points of the carotid arteries. To do this, place your fingertips at the angle of your jaw just below the ear lobes; now bring them down an inch or two and you should be able to feel the pulsation of the carotid arteries. Do not press too hard or too long on a carotid artery. Feel first one carotid pulse and then the other, and compare the strength of the two. They should be approximately equal. A carotid pulse that seems markedly weaker than the other may indicate a narrowing of that carotid artery. This is an important finding that your doctor should know about.

3. Finally, take your stethoscope and listen to the carotid arteries. Following the instructions for the use of the stethoscope given in Chapter 1, place the chest piece on the carotid pulse. Be sure to hold your breath while you listen or you will hear great, loud rushes of air each time you take a breath.

Normally, you should hear nothing at all when you listen to the carotid pulse using a stethoscope; if anything, you may hear your heart beating faintly in the distance. Should there be an area of constriction somewhere along the artery, however, the flow of blood through the vessel will make a whooshing sound. Doctors call this a *bruit,* which is simply French for noise. If you think you hear this whooshing sound and you are sure it's not just the sound of your breathing, you should have your suspicions checked out by a doctor.

CHAPTER 8

IDENTIFYING AND TRACKING SKIN BLEMISHES AND AILMENTS

The skin is the great envelope that wraps the body; it is our largest organ, comprising 15 percent of our body weight, and it is the most visible aspect of ourselves that we present to the outside world. So we pamper our skin, worry over it and bemoan every spot that detracts from its loveliness. We worry so much about our skin, in fact, that severe, widespread blemishing, such as occurs in acne or psoriasis, can cause marked personality changes in its victims.

Trauma that destroys as little as 10 percent of the skin covering the body has serious medical consequences, and if something more than half the skin is damaged by burns or other injury, the chance of death, even with careful management, becomes substantial.

Consider how many functions the skin performs:

- Skin is a protective shield and a waterproof overcoat for the body. Skin prevents noxious elements in the environment from getting at more delicate tissues underneath. Skin pigment protects us from the damaging effects of ultraviolet rays from the sun.
- Skin prevents loss of vital fluids and other substances from within the body.
- Skin is a thermal shield and helps in the regulation and maintenance of body temperature.
- Skin is an excretory organ, helping to rid the body of excess water and waste materials.
- Skin contains nerves that enable us to feel through touch and alert us to danger from invasion or changes in temperature.
- Skin is a factory that produces essential vitamin D.

We use our skin extensively in nonverbal communication of our emotions: we wrinkle the skin in different ways to express joy or sorrow, worry or anger; the skin blushes with embarrassment and blanches with shock or fear. Skin is an identification factor in its color and in the distinctive patterns it forms on the hands and feet; it tells our age and sometimes gives us a characteristic odor. Skin and hair are sexually attractive; skin touching is sexually stimulating, comforting, and reassuring. And the appearance of the skin can provide important information about the general state of one's health.

Rashes occur with many illnesses that affect the body systems—measles, chickenpox, and secondary syphilis are among these. Chronic itching may herald anything from nervousness to serious disease. Discoloration of the skin may point to disease—yellowing in jaundice and darkening in Addison's disease. Excessive and inappropriate sweating can result from simple nervousness, drugs, alcohol, or a hormonal imbalance. Sweating on one side of the body only may tell of nerve or brain damage, while hot, dry skin can tell of fever or sunstroke.

You may have noticed that one of the first things a doctor does in performing a general examination is to take your hands and gently look first at one side and then the other. He will rather caressingly run his hand over your arm and perhaps your back. This does two things—it calms you and establishes rapport through touching, and it provides a wealth of information about you and your general physical condition.

THE STRUCTURE OF THE SKIN

The skin is composed of several layers. The top layer, called the epidermis, is the part most often thought of as being typical skin. It has two main types of cells, keratinocytes and melanocytes. The keratinocytes produce a special material called keratin which is a system of threadlike filaments imbedded in a nonstructured, gluey substance. This gives the skin toughness that enables it to withstand a good deal of pounding and scraping.

The other important cell type in the epidermis is the melanocyte. These cells produce pigment, called melanin, and, as you might expect, people with dark skins have a large number of active melanocytes whereas people with fair skins have few or inactive cells of this type. Tanning after exposure to the sun is due to increased amounts of melanin in the skin.

The second layer of the skin is called the dermis. This is filled with a variety of structures that serve the skin and the rest of the body in a number of ways. There is connective tissue that gives strength and resiliency to the skin, blood vessels that nourish skin cells and that carry waste materials to the skin to be disposed of, nerves that detect touch and temperature change, oil glands, sweat glands, hair follicles, and tiny muscles.

The epidermis and the dermis lie atop a layer of fat which is sometimes called the subcutaneous tissue (meaning "under the skin") that acts as a cushion and shock absorber for the skin and separates it from the underlying muscle and bone. Skin can be as much as one-quarter inch thick over the soles of the feet, or as thin as one-fiftieth inch over the eyelids and the eardrum. The subcutaneous fatty tissue adds thickness in most places around the body with the exception of such sites as the shins and the outer shells of the ears where you can feel bone and cartilage directly underneath the skin.

The outermost cells of the epidermis, called the stratum corneum, or horny layer, are actually dead cells that constantly dry and fall off. These cells are replaced by others that migrate to the surface from underneath in a process which goes on continually. New cells are produced at the bottom of the epidermis and slowly die, flatten out, and move to the surface of the skin. The full cycle takes a little less than a month, which means that you replace the outer layer of the skin about twelve times a year. This process is highly visible when you see the outer surface of the skin peel in large flakes after having been burned by the sun. Both hair and fingernails, incidentally, are made up of these dead epidermal cells that have undergone specialized changes.

EXAMINING YOUR SKIN
AND TRACKING SKIN HEALTH

Dermatology is the medical specialty which deals with disorders of the skin. The dermatologist depends mostly upon keen powers of observation and extensive training in recognizing several hundred kinds of skin disorders. So most tests for skin disease are simply very close observations of the nature of the lesion being dealt with. A detailed medical history and close questioning about a person's habits and environment are also essential ingredients that go into a dermatologist's diagnosis. Sometimes the dermatologist uses a magnifying glass to help see the exact structure of a lesion; he may arrange his examining lights to either create or eliminate shadows, and he may use a long-wave ultraviolet light called a Wood's light which helps in detecting fungus infections and some disorders of skin pigment.

The dermatologist also uses the laboratory, either sending skin scrapings out for analysis, or making on-the-spot microscopic exami-

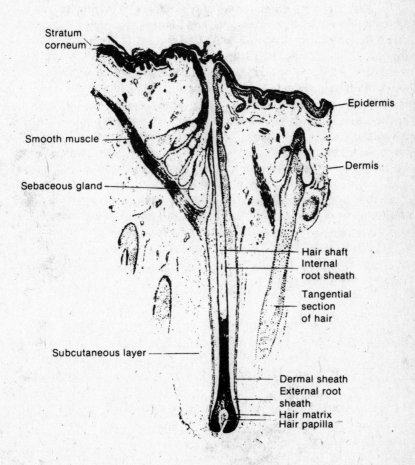

Structures of the Skin

nations. The dermatologist frequently resorts to skin biopsies for diagnosis of suspicious lesions. This is done by applying a local anesthetic and then taking a circle of skin, including part of the lesion, with a little round cutting tool called a biopsy punch. This sample is then sent to a pathology laboratory for examination. A normal complement of blood tests is also used in diagnosing some skin problems.

Because similar skin disorders may originate in the environment, in a person's system due to generalized disease, or even in a person's mind, the process of diagnosis will often challenge the imagination of a Sherlock Holmes and the wisdom of a Solomon. Treatment may be as simple as changing an irritating laundry detergent or as complicated as managing a broadside of medications. Obviously, then, an untrained person cannot do the job of a dermatologist for himself or for anyone else. But it is definitely useful and sometimes can be lifesaving to know your skin and to keep track of what it is doing. So part of your health-tracking procedure should include close, systematic observation of your skin, and records should be kept of your skin condition and the location and size of any blemishes.

To do a skin examination you will have to work with a partner since most skin areas are where you can't see them easily by yourself. Mirrors can help in a self-examination but they don't allow the careful observations you need to make.

Examining the Skin

1. The examiner should follow an orderly routine so as not to miss anything. Begin with the hands—palms, backs, fingernails, and between the fingers. Then proceed from the top down—hair and scalp, face and neck, shoulders, trunk and arms, and so on. Be sure to check skin folds, armpits, the groin area, genitals, and other hidden places which provide exceptionally fine growing conditions for bacteria and fungi.

2. Make notes as you go. The examiner may talk into a tape recorder nearby or the subject may take down notes as the examiner makes observations.

3. Try to notice and comment upon everything, no matter how usual or insignificant it may seem. If you miss something such as "cool, dry palms," it may not seem unusual later if the palms change to moist and clammy.

4. Some things you should notice include:

   • Condition of the skin: rough, smooth, dry, oily, flaking
   • Color: pale, flushed, uniform or nonuniform
   • Marks, irregularities and blemishes: bumps and lumps, moles, freckles, warts, age spots, sores, discolorations, bleeding or

crusting, unexplained black and blue marks. Note the size, color, and how long the subject has had the mark or sore. Measure blemishes with a small ruler, preferably one that is calibrated in millimeters. Use a hand magnifying glass to accurately describe the color, nature, and texture of blemishes.
- Note complaints of chronic itching, evidence of scratch marks, complaints of profuse sweating when there is no apparent reason for it.

Once you are aware of everything that is on your skin it is both interesting and informative to have all of your observations explained. With notes and questions in hand, visit a dermatologist, have your skin examined professionally, and have him or her explain your collection of lumps, bumps, and blemishes. At this time you can find out which are not worth worrying about and which you should keep an eye on. You may also find that some annoying blemishes can be easily gotten rid of.

It is not a waste of time and money to visit a doctor—even a specialist—when you are well. Specialists are so used to seeing patients only when they are in trouble that the doctor may wonder at your initiative, but once you explain your interest you are likely to be well received. Then once you have an intelligent record, any disturbing changes that occur can be evaluated and treated quickly.

A change in a mole or a change in other blemishes is especially important and one of the American Cancer Society's cardinal signs of skin cancer. Melanoma, a particularly insidious and virulent form of skin cancer, often starts out from slightly raised skin lesions such as a mole or an age spot, and in the course of enlarging changes from a medium to a dark brown to a bluish or dark gray color. But any skin blemish that changes in size, color, or texture should be evaluated professionally without delay.

Skin cancers are among the most common malignancies found in people and the killer potential of melanoma can't be emphasized too strongly. Early diagnosis, which means early discovery, followed by removal of the malignancy is lifesaving. Once the malignancy begins to spread from its original site there is no satisfactory treatment at this time and death rates are high. Prospects for cure are excellent, on the other hand, with early diagnosis and removal.

Danger Signs of Malignancy in a Pigmented (Colored) Blemish

1. The appearance of varying colors should be viewed with sus-

picion. When colors such as red, white, or blue appear in any skin blemish, it must be investigated.

2. If the border of a skin blemish becomes irregular, especially with noticeable notching at some point, it is suggestive of trouble.

3. When the surface of a blemish becomes irregular, bumpy, rough, and uneven, a developing melanoma may be suspected.

FOR YOUR PERSONAL HEALTH RECORD

1. Record the general appearance and condition of the skin. There may be something special to note about one part of the body—condition of the scalp and hair, appearance of fingernails and toenails, roughness or flaking on the legs, and so on.

2. Note the location, size, color, and texture of skin blemishes. If there are many moles, make a sketch that locates most of them.

3. Record any chronic complaints of itching, recurrent sores, fever blisters, boils, warts, and so on.

4. Record the date and repeat the examination every six months. Compare subsequent examinations with previous ones for significant differences that should be discussed with your doctor.

The diagnosis and treatment of skin disorders is an extremely complicated business. Many conditions have similar appearances and their causes are frequently difficult to ascertain and are often unknown. Therefore, any unusual eruptions should be called to the attention of a doctor. Because skin disorders can have causes other than skin dysfunction, other specialists besides a dermatologist are sometimes needed. Internists, allergists, the specialist in family medicine, and at times the help of a psychiatrist may be called upon.

The blemishes and disorders described in this chapter are only a sampling of the woes a person's skin may fall heir to, but because they are the most common ones you should have at least a passing acquaintance with them.

BLEMISHES AND VARIATIONS ON NORMAL SKIN

Moles.   Moles usually begin as flat brown spots and then become slightly raised. They are simply clusters of melanocytes, the normal skin cells that produce pigment, and more than 95 percent of adults have them. In areas of normal white skin, melanocytes are widely scattered and produce only small amounts of pigment. It is the clustering of these cells that produces the characteristic brown color of moles.

The reason that people are cautioned to watch moles for changes is that melanoma, the virulent skin cancer mentioned earlier, originates in melanocytes. Because there are melanocytes all over the body, melanoma can originate anywhere, with or without a mole. But because moles are concentrations of melanocytes, the chances of a melanoma beginning in a mole are somewhat increased over other skin areas. A mole that does not show signs of changing, and that has been pronounced safe in the course of a regular examination, may safely be left alone unless you want it removed for cosmetic reasons.

Hemangiomas (Birthmarks).   Red patches on the skin may be present at birth or appear in the first year or so of a baby's life.

"Stork bite" is a name given to little pink or salmon-colored patches that appear on the eyelids, the forehead, or the nape of the neck of newborns and fade away spontaneously in a few months or a year.

"Port-wine stain" can also be present at birth. It is a flat patch, colored red or purple-red, and may enlarge over the first few months before stabilizing. Except for the coloring, the skin is normal and rarely presents anything but a cosmetic problem. Occasionally a port-wine stain indicates a blood-vessel abnormality, but your pediatrician will be aware of this and will advise you accordingly. Port-wine stains do not fade and at the present time nothing can be done about them. If they are in a noticeable place cosmetic covering creams can help somewhat.

"Strawberry marks" may be present at birth but they appear more frequently during the first month of life. They tend to be bright red and are raised. They may grow rapidly for a while, but then the majority of them disappear by themselves over a period of several years.

All of these red markings are caused by a large collection of capillaries (tiny blood vessels) under the skin, so you can check rather easily to see if a red mark you are looking at is one of these:

Identifying Hemangiomas

1. Press down on the mark with a clear piece of glass you can see through. An ordinary water glass or wine glass will do.

2. Hold for a few seconds and observe the mark through the glass. If there is some blanching of the red mark where you press down, you are looking at an area of skin that is filled with tiny blood vessels—a

hemangioma. Your doctor can tell you for sure what kind it is and what you may expect in terms of its staying or going away.

3. If the color does not blanch when you press down, it is probably a small bruise.

Liver Spots and Freckles.   Liver spots, or lentigines, are similar to moles in that there are increased numbers of melanocytes that produce a characteristic brown to black color. But these cells don't cluster as they do in moles and so liver spots remain small and flat. They mostly inhabit the face and the backs of the hands and are probably related to exposure to the sun in the course of a lifetime. They are characteristic of aging but may appear early in life as well. Sun worshipers and people who work outdoors are likely to develop more liver spots earlier than people whose skin is protected from the sun most of the time.

The tendency to have freckles is inherited and they seem to result more from highly active melanocytes than from clusters of them. After exposure to the sun the melanocytes become large and very active, increasing the amount of pigment in the freckle spots.

Melasma.   This frequently occurs in pregnant women or in those who are taking oral contraceptives, but the condition is also found on occasion in men, as well as in women who are not pregnant and not using oral contraceptives. It seems especially common among Latin people.

Melasma is a darkening of skin pigment in patches about the face and is strictly of temporary cosmetic concern because no other symptoms are involved and the patches of skin eventually return to their normal color. A dermatologist can usually manage to lighten the darkened areas gradually so that when the condition disappears the skin will return to its normal color. Permanent skin bleaches should be avoided because these simply cause the opposite problem—white patches.

Vitiligo.   Loss of skin pigment in patches that leave white areas of skin with sharply defined borders is called vitiligo. It is most commonly a genetic disorder that appears in families in an irregular inheritance pattern. For reasons that are presently unknown, the melanocytes in patches of the skin completely disappear. These patches may be tiny and barely noticeable or may involve large portions of the body.

A few other things can account for loss of skin color: injury, burns, certain fungus infections, and glandular diseases; but you are likely to know about an injury or infection, and a glandular disease will make itself known with other symptoms of illness.

Seborrheic Keratosis.   This is a benign skin tumor that resembles a mole but becomes thicker and often looks like it has been stuck onto the skin. It may feel oily or rough and dry. These lesions seldom appear before age forty, and when large numbers of them occur it may turn out to be a family trait. They are not harmful, but if they present a cosmetic problem or if they are a nuisance for some other reason they can easily be removed by a doctor.

Skin Tags.   Skin tags are little protrusions or polyps of normally colored skin. They resemble little nipples and may appear about the eyelids, the neck, and the trunk and in upper-body creases that occur with obesity. Skin tags are harmless and may be left alone, but if they are a bother they can be removed quite easily by a doctor.

Benign Cysts and Tumors.   Lumps and swellings covered by normally colored skin may occur in any of the skin layers or in the fatty, subcutaneous tissue. These are known as dermatofibromas, wens, and lipomas. Any such lumps should be investigated by a doctor. If it is indeed one of the structures mentioned it is no cause for concern and the doctor will probably leave it up to you as to whether you want it removed or not. However, if one is growing in a place where it might become a cosmetic problem in the future or interfere with wearing certain kinds of clothing, it is probably a good idea to have it removed sooner than later so that the resulting scar can be a small one.

IRRITATIONS, INJURIES, AND SENSITIVITIES

Diaper Rash.   Called napkin rash by those who call diapers napkins, this is the first skin irritation that most of us experience, and it is caused by the irritating effects of urine and feces held against the skin by the diaper. The entire diaper area becomes red and inflamed, and baby will usually let you know just how uncomfortable it feels. Pimples, sores, and blisters may also occur. Strict cleanliness is essential—which means not just frequent diaper changes but frequent rinsing as well. Tight rubber pants or plastic diaper coverings worn for long periods should be avoided. Frequent air drying of skin is a good idea, and if you use cloth reusable diapers they should not be laundered in harsh soaps. When the irritation is severe a doctor should be consulted.

Sunburn.   Sunburn is caused by middle-length ultraviolet rays of the sun—which you do not feel—not by the infrared rays which feel warm on the skin. So you may burn without feeling warm on a cloudy day and feel warm without burning if you take your sun under glass, which screens out the ultraviolet rays but admits the infrared.

Sunburn results in injury to the skin. The skin defends itself by increasing its rate of growth to replace damaged skin (resulting in peeling), and by producing extra melanin (pigment) to screen out further attacks of ultraviolet radiation, which manifests itself as tanning. Chronic exposure to the ultraviolet rays of the sun over the years contributes to early skin wrinkling and to more, larger, and darker liver spots.

It is quite well established that development of skin cancer has direct links to sun exposure. Skin cancer occurs most frequently in fair people, in people who work in the sun, and in people who play in the sun, and it most often occurs on sun-exposed areas of the skin.

Sunscreen lotions are better than nothing when you are out in the sun because they block out some ultraviolet light, but most are inefficient. If they blocked out all the ultraviolet rays, people using them would not tan at all and would not buy them. Then, too, lotions quickly wash off with sweating or swimming, and they rub off just by your turning on a beach blanket.

Heat and Chemical Burns.   Fire, scalding water, and abrasive chemicals cause direct and instantaneous injury. These burns are classified according to the depth of the injury and the amount of damage done to the various skin tissues:

First-degree burns. Surface skin is hurt but living skin cells are not damaged. There is pain, redness, and perhaps some swelling. This burn heals by itself in a few days.

Second-degree burns. Here, in addition to pain and redness there is blistering and weeping of fluid. Living epidermal cells just below the surface skin are killed, but the epidermal layer remains largely intact and will rebuild itself within a month or less without scarring.

Since it is not always easy to tell the difference between second- and third-degree burns, even for a physician, any serious burn as large as an inch or more should be shown to a doctor. There is always danger of infection.

Third-degree burns. Third-degree burns completely destroy cells of the epidermal layer so that new skin cannot be regenerated at the burn site and scarring will result. The deeper dermal layer and even the fatty tissue underneath may be destroyed. The skin will probably look charred or otherwise eroded. There may not be pain immediately if nerve endings have been destroyed. These are always serious and skin grafting is usually necessary for proper healing.

When extremely severe burns have been sustained, as when someone has been taken from a burning building or subjected to extensive scalding, you can assume third-degree burns have occurred and expert help should be sought at once. Kitchen burns, when they occur quickly and there is no prolonged contact with a hot surface, flame, superheated fat, or scalding water, are usually first or second degree. Sunburn is generally a first-degree burn, but prolonged exposure of sensitive skin can result in the blistering and swelling of second-degree burns. Chemical burns can continue to increase in severity if the irritating substance is not thoroughly flushed away from the skin.

Third-degree burns must be managed with the utmost of expert care, especially if they are extensive. They can be life-threatening. When the skin covering is removed, the body loses fluids in great quantities and it is laid open to the most massive and dangerous infections.

Dry Skin. Everyone knows about dry skin from watching television commercials, and each of us has a favorite remedy for the problem that may range in price from a few cents to many dollars depending on how many "secret" or "mysterious" ingredients are claimed for the product. But then the earliest records of humankind tell of people annointing themselves with oils, so we must assume that the TV generation is not the first to suffer from dry skin.

Dry skin is dehydration of the surface layer of the skin, which means that water present there naturally has evaporated. Skin tends to be more dry as we age. Domestic and commercial cleaners and solvents remove oils from the skin that help retain moisture, and the skin dries. Wet skin swells and becomes soft while dry skin shrinks and becomes brittle. So when you have your hands in and out of water constantly the skin may crack and roughen from the continual changes.

Dry skin feels dry. It may be rough and it may peel or flake. There is itching and the consequent scratching makes things worse. Eczema or secondary infection can result from scratching and an itch-scratch cycle can develop.

Treatment for dry skin consists of allowing the water that is naturally present in the skin to stay there. You don't have to "moisturize" your skin, the skin does that by itself. Use an oil to hold in skin moisture (hand cream, bath oil, petroleum jelly) and avoid excess soap and other drying agents. If general drying of body skin is a problem, humidifying the atmosphere in winter with a room humidifier will help.

Itching.   Sometimes the cause of itching is obvious, sometimes it is not. Chemical irritants, dryness, sweating, rough clothing can all cause itching. Sensitivity to certain foods or drugs and some systemic diseases cause itching. The list is endless. Rapid temperature changes can cause skin to itch, and nervousness, puzzlement, or confusion can start an itch going. If you are bothered with itching it may get worse at night in a warm bed when you have more time to think about it.

The natural response to itching is rubbing or scratching. Persistent rubbing and scratching can cause a dermatitis that requires more scratching and the itch-scratch cycle begins. In some cases the itch-scratch cycle is so severe that an angry infection results.

Careful inquiry and detective work is usually needed to find the cause of itching where the reason is not obvious, and this is one of those times when a well-kept medical history can pay off. Records of medicines, diet, chronic disorders, life style, temperament, may all provide clues for your doctor.

Hives.   A temporary swelling in the dermal layer of the skin results in a hive—which is sort of a giant mosquito bite. The swelling is often caused by a histamine, a protein released in response to sensitivity or allergy to some substance. Finding the allergy or source of sensitivity can involve a bit of detective work or the cause may be obvious—an insect bite, a drug just taken, or the observation that hives occur every time you eat a certain food. Stress and nervousness seem to bring them out on some people. When hives are severe an antihistamine may be prescribed to combat the histamines present. If the onset of hives follows taking a prescribed drug, the doctor should be informed at once since they may herald a more serious reaction later.

Contact Dermatitis.   This is a skin eruption caused by some irritant—industrial chemicals or poison ivy, for example. If you are allergic or sensitive to a substance with which you come in contact, an eczema can develop within one to three days.

Once again a careful history and a bit of detective work is needed to discover and remove the offending substance. Were you out of doors and exposed to poison ivy in the last few days? What other substances have you been exposed to? The site of the irritation may be revealing. Eczema on the wrist or finger may identify a watch, bracelet, or ring as the culprit (even if the jewelry is of a high-karat gold). Blisters in streaky lines on arms or legs point to poison ivy because the plant's irritating oil tends to streak across the skin as you brush against it.

If poison ivy or other contact dermatitis is severe, it is a problem for the special skills of a dermatologist.

ECZEMA AND DERMATITIS

The words *eczema* and *dermatitis* are very general words used to refer to many kinds of skin ailments. Dermatitis simply means an inflammation of the skin. Eczema describes a series of events that occur on the skin: redness, swelling, the appearance of small, fluid-filled vesicles (tiny blisters), oozing, scaling, and crusting. To say that you have a dermatitis simply means that you have a skin irritation of some kind that has not yet been described precisely. To say that you have eczema means that the skin has gotten a bit messy-looking as a result of something that is wrong with it. There are many causes of eczema and dermatitis, some of which are well known and others that are unknown and puzzling. Following are some of the most common that you are liable to see.

Acne Vulgaris.   The pimples, blackheads, nodules, cysts, and scars of acne are too well known to need describing. They occur on the face, neck, shoulders, and back, and when it occurs it seems to be a body response to hormone changes during puberty. Arising in the teen years it may persist into the late twenties or even the thirties. It is one of the many skin ailments that are poorly understood. The term *vulgaris* added to the medical name simply means it is a very common form of acne, not vulgar in the sense that we commonly use the word.

It is known that acne is not caused by dirty habits, masturbation, chocolate, greasy foods, or any other identifiable teenage indulgence. On the other hand, it is also known that parental pressure, guilt feelings, social self-consciousness, stress, and tension may precipitate flare-ups.

While the cause of acne is unknown and there is neither cure nor preventive at this time, there have been tremendous strides made in treating acne so that improvement in one's appearance can be attained in nearly every case. But acne sufferers should be under the care of a competent dermatologist because a carefully managed program of antibiotics and skin care is often required. Unsupervised home treatment is usually worse than useless. Denying a young person access to care by a competent dermatologist on the assumption that he or she will "outgrow it" is cruel and can lead to scarring that could have been prevented.

Seborrheic Dermatitis.   This is yet another dermatitis of unknown cause.

Seborrheic dermatitis appears as a red, scaly eruption in the same areas as acne—face, chest, and back—and in addition may invade the scalp. It may first appear in infancy, then disappear and then return again after puberty and persist all during adult life.

Like so many skin disorders, emotional stress seems to play some mysterious role in recurrences. Dermatologists can treat the symptoms with some success and bring relief to those affected, but there is no cure at the present time.

Psoriasis.   Approximately six million people in the United States have psoriasis. No one suffering from psoriasis should restrict himself to patent preparations but should seek professional help. While psoriasis cannot be cured, under the direction of a good dermatologist it is eminently treatable; lesions can be reduced and flare-ups can be minimized.

Psoriasis manifests itself as clusters of slightly raised, scablike plaques which occur most often in bony places such as the knees and elbows. The lesions can occur anywhere on the body, however, and when they are widespread they can be both demoralizing and debilitating.

Hand Eczemas.   Both at home and in the industrial world hand eczema is the most common skin ailment. When your hands are constantly exposed to drying and irritating agents, as they are in homemaking and many other occupations, some or all of the events that take the name eczema can occur—redness, swelling, the appearnce of tiny blisters, oozing, scaling, and crusting. For want of better names, hand eczemas may be designated as dishpan hands, bartender's hands, laboratory hands, and so on, depending on the source of the irritation. Diagnosis is usually made by taking a careful history and doing laboratory tests to eliminate other possible causes of the eczema.

Heat Rash or Prickly Heat.   This happens when sweat ducts become obstructed.

Look for redness and a rash composed of tiny red bumps or small blisters. The condition and the rash become worse with sweating. Looking at the skin with a magnifying glass you will find that the little bumps or blisters are at sweat pores but never at a pore where there is a hair growing.

Anything that helps prevent sweating is helpful—air conditioning, well-ventilated clothing, and so on.

Pityriasis Rosea.   Another skin disorder of unknown cause or origin. (Doctors say "A disease of uncertain etiology," which means "We haven't cracked this one yet." And, as you may have noticed, there are many of these in the realm of dermatology.) This mysterious ailment, however, disappears by itself within about eight weeks as mysteriously as it appears.

Pityriasis rosea is a rash consisting of small pink or red circles that have a collar of scales around the edge. The center of the lesion may be clear or just a bit crinkly or wrinkled. The rash often has a characteristic distribution of sort of arching lines that go from the ears to the hips, and when viewed from the back with some imagination the pattern may seem to form a crude picture of a fir tree—a Christmas tree. It is often preceded by a "herald patch" or blotch elsewhere on the body.

Diagnosis is usually made by seeing what the lesions look like under a magnifying glass, by observing the fir-tree distribution of lesions, and by the fact that other tests performed by the doctor prove negative.

SKIN INFECTIONS

The skin is alive with microorganisms—bacteria, viruses, yeasts, and fungi. Sometimes, under certain circumstances, there are small animals such as mites and insects. Most of this wildlife lives on the skin because it is a hospitable environment with plenty of moisture and warmth, innumerable cracks and crannies to hide in, and lots of food in the form of dead skin and body excretions. Practically all these organisms are harmless and some actually help us by keeping down populations of potentially harmful bacteria.

There are some villains, however, that will invade the skin or even

invade the body *through* the skin when they get an opportunity. These
cause a variety of infections. Following are some of the most common.

Boils.   Most people have experienced boils on occasion, but there
are some people who are apparently susceptible to them and get them
rather often. A boil is a local infection caused by a staphylococcus
bacterium and may arise anywhere on the body; a sty, for example, is a
boil on the eyelid.

A boil starts out as a red bump that enlarges slowly until it is as
much as ½ inch or 1½ inches across. There is often throbbing pain or
burning. After several days the boil becomes soft and pus-filled. A
yellow or white head appears in the middle on its surface. If left alone it
will eventually rupture, drain itself of a mixture of pus and blood, and
begin to heal.

It is best to have a boil seen and treated by a doctor, especially if it is
large, if you get them frequently, or if several appear at the same time.
Puncturing or squeezing a boil while it is still hard may make the
infection worse. Once the boil is draining it should be kept clean and
covered with a dressing. The staphylococcus bacteria are highly infectious, so until the boil heals, scrupulous cleanliness and careful dis-
posal of dressings should be rigorously enforced.

Medically, a boil is called a furuncle. A carbuncle is several
furuncles that connect with each other in the dermal layer of the skin
and in the fatty subcutaneous tissue. These are large and painful areas
that may persist for as much as two weeks before coming to a head.
There may be some fever with carbuncles. They should always be seen
and treated by a physician, never treated with home remedies.

Impetigo.   This is usually thought of as a disease of small children, and indeed it is seen most frequently among infants and youngsters, but anyone can get impetigo. Once again, streptococcus bacteria are usually the culprits, although sometimes more than one kind
of bacteria is present.

Impetigo starts with a flat area of redness and then tiny blisters
develop which break, ooze, and form a brown or yellow crust. It may
go away by itself eventually, but spreading and complications are more
often the rule if professional help is not sought promptly.

Ringworm.   Ringworm is not a worm but a fungus infection
whose lesions are roughly ring-shaped. These fungi have a special
taste for dead skin, hair, and nails—it's all they eat. Poor hygiene and

poor living conditions increase the chances of contracting ringworm, but anyone can get it.

Ringworm of the body is usually flat, scaly, and red. The center of the ring clears as the scaly red edge advances.

Ringworm of the scalp produces round, sharply outlined areas where hairs are broken off just above the skin. The lesions may be light and flaky, but they may also be moist and badly inflamed. Both body and scalp ringworm are most common in children and may become epidemic among children who congregate together.

Ringworm of the feet (athlete's foot) affects at least half the adults in the United States at some time during their lives. The fungus is found anywhere that feet go. It causes minor scaling and cracking between the toes, but if left unattended it can spread widely and become badly inflamed. Then, secondary infection can occur.

Ringworm of the groin (jock itch) occurs most often in men and may be carried to the groin from affected feet.

Any infection of ringworm should be seen by a doctor so that both the disease and the specific organism causing it can be positively identified and proper treatment can be prescribed.

Warts.   Most people are familiar with these rough, flesh-colored bumps that frequently turn up on the hands. And anyone who has read *Tom Sawyer* knows how to cure warts: You stick the hand with the warts in water gathered in an old stump and say, "Spunk water, spunk water, swallow these warts."

The funny thing about warts is that this and a hundred other folklore remedies often work in getting rid of them even though it has been clearly established that warts are caused by a virus. The point is that warts seem to be psychosuggestible for reasons that are not yet understood. In laboratory experiments doctors have "cured" warts with treatments as bizarre and as obviously worthless as spunk water. And, using suggestion, they have been able to make a patient's warts disappear on one hand and remain on the other. Warts may also disappear without treatment and without suggestion.

There are, however, many simple and reliable medical cures for warts, so your best bet in dealing with them is to show them to a doctor, especially if you have many of them or get them frequently.

Warts have different names and slightly different appearances depending upon where they occur:

Finger warts are generally flesh-colored, rough, and may have black dots scattered through them.

Face warts, neck, or shoulder warts may be shaped like little fingers.

Plantar warts grow on the bottom of the foot and tend to grow inward because of the pressure of standing and walking on them. They can become quite painful.

Soft, nonhorny warts that look something like tiny cauliflowers may appear in moist areas—the armpits, groin, anus, and vagina. These are sometimes called venereal warts although they can be acquired in other ways besides sexual contact.

Herpes Simplex.   The herpes virus is best known for causing fever blisters (cold sores) about the mouth, but it may invade the skin anywhere, or the mucous membranes inside the mouth, the eyes, or the genitals, where it can produce angry infections.

Herpes simplex skin infections usually show up as clusters of tiny blisters which may be mixed with pimples. These ooze and form crusts, and there is often swelling and redness.

On mucous membranes of the mouth or genitals, herpes simplex appears as a cluster of pitted sores surrounded by a red, inflamed-looking area.

Herpes infections are recurrent in some people. Fever blisters about the mouth, for example, may come and go at the same site several times a year. There is no preventive and no known cure at this time, but if an infection is extensive or painful, symptoms should be treated by a doctor to bring as much relief as possible and to avoid secondary infections. Herpes infections around the eyes can endanger eyesight and should be seen by a doctor at once.

Canker Sores.   Canker sores occur only in the mucous membrane lining of the mouth. They are similar in appearance to herpes simplex but they are not caused by the herpes virus. It is not known, in fact, what causes canker sores and there is no treatment except to alleviate pain and try to prevent secondary infections. The sores heal in a week or ten days and they tend to recur at the same sites in people who get them. Dentists working with college students have reported seeing small epidemics of canker sores that coincide with exam time.

Skin Ulcers.   A skin ulcer might better be called a nasty-looking sore. Ulcers result from causes as obvious as an injury, or they may result from something more obscure, such as poor circulation in the legs, diabetes, a malignancy, or syphilis.

If a skin ulcer appears that can't be explained by an injury, or if a sore persists and becomes worse instead of healing quickly, it should be shown to a doctor without delay. If a painless ulcer appears in the groin area, especially on the genitals, on the mouth or tongue, breast or nipples, syphilis may be suspected as a possible cause. (A more detailed discussion of the signs of syphilis can be found below where we discuss systemic disorders that show on the skin.)

Ulcers which appear on the lower parts of the legs, on the ankles or feet, and that persist or recur, are usually due to poor circulation in veins or arteries. This is most often seen in older people. The sore is likely to begin as a painful red spot which becomes blue or purplish. The skin then breaks down to form an ulcer.

Lice and Scabies.   While the infections we have been talking about are caused by invading microorganisms, lice and scabies are infestations of small parasitic insects. Lice are tiny, bloodsucking insects, while scabies are even tinier, spiderlike animals that burrow under the skin.

Lice live on body hairs or in clothing and venture forth from time to time to get a meal of blood. Itching is severe and eggs and developing lice can be found attached to a hair or a thread of clothing.

Crab lice are a variety of body lice that inhabit the pubic area. They are smaller than body lice and are harder to see with the naked eye. Under a magnifying glass they are seen to have little pincers that make them look like crabs and hence their name.

In scabies the female mite burrows under the skin to lay eggs. There is severe itching, often just at bedtime, and you can see red lines on the skin where the mite has done its burrowing. The doctor will treat both lice and scabies by prescribing a pesticide and will check for any infection that may have been caused by scratching. Then, clothing and bedclothes must be scrupulously laundered.

A word of caution: All skin infections should be handled cautiously to prevent spreading the infection to others or to other parts of the body. Extra special care should be taken not to transfer microorganisms from a skin infection to a skin area that is injured (scratched, for example) or already raw from another ailment.

Most skin ailments are not contagious, however, and it is quite disturbing psychologically for a person with a noninfectious skin ailment to have others shrink away from him. Acne is not contagious, and neither are psoriasis or vitiligo. People with these ailments should be given the reassurance of touching by their families.

SYSTEMIC DISEASES THAT SHOW ON THE SKIN

A number of ailments that affect the body systems—and so are usually called systemic diseases—may affect the skin as well. People in good health, especially children, have an unmistakable glow about them that bespeaks their well-being. Pallor, flushing, dryness, unreasonable sweating, rashes, all speak of something wrong going on inside that should be investigated.

When a systemic disease is present, such as measles, scarlet fever, or chicken pox, there is first a general feeling of malaise, fever, and so on, and then a characteristic rash appears on the skin. Skin lesions are the only outward signs of the presence of early syphilis. Drugs you are allergic to may cause skin eruptions. Following are brief descriptions of some common systemic ailments that show themselves on the skin.

Syphilis. The corkscrew-shaped spirochete that causes syphilis can penetrate intact, healthy skin, and within hours it enters the bloodstream. So syphilis can be said to be a systemic disease from the outset.

In a little more than a week, or as much as a month after the initial infection, one sore, called a chancre, will appear on the skin at the site where the spirochetes entered—on the genitals, mouth parts, or elsewhere depending on how sexual contact was made with the affected partner. And, incidentally, it may not be obvious that a partner has syphilis in an infectious stage.

The chancre is painless, round, slightly raised, and has a hard base that may feel as if there is a nickel or a dime buried under the skin. Left alone the chancre will heal in 30 to 90 days, but the spirochetes remain and continue to multiply and circulate in the bloodstream. This is primary syphilis.

The next episode, secondary syphilis, results from a systemwide reaction to the bacteria. This appears on the skin as a generalized rash involving all skin surfaces, even the palms of the hands and the soles of the feet and the mucous lining of the mouth. The nature of the rash may vary from one individual to the next but an identifying feature is that all skin marks appear the same—all red and flat, all raised and scaly, all red bumps, and so on. Whenever a doctor sees a generalized, uniform rash that shows lesions on the palms and soles, he suspects syphilis until he can prove otherwise through blood tests.

The rash, too, disappears and the syphilis becomes latent for a number of years. When it next turns up it may affect any part of the body. Some favorite sites are the central nervous system, the heart, and arteries leading to the heart.

The greatest danger from syphilis comes from ignoring early symptoms because they are painless and disappear spontaneously. It is a most serious disease at any stage, and even a suspicion that it exists should be enough to send you to a physician for diagnosis and treatment if necessary.

Drug Eruption.   When any skin eruption—rash, redness, hives, or whatever—appears while you are taking any drug, even aspirin, the drug should be suspected as one possible cause of the skin problem. And when drugs are suspected, the person's general condition should be monitored carefully on the chance that the skin eruption is heralding a more serious allergic reaction. If a doctor has administered the drug, he or she should be notified at once of the reaction.

Measles, Chicken Pox, and Scarlet Fever.   Measles is a serious disease and too often a deadly one. Children can be immunized against measles and should be. If the disease does appear, however, a doctor should always be consulted.

The measles rash is purplish-red and as a general rule first appears in the head area—on the forehead, behind the ears, and on the neck. It then spreads to involve the whole body. The small spots are flat (not raised) and as new ones appear further down the body the old ones tend to merge together to become big, splashy spots. A cough may precede the appearance of spots on the skin and if the throat is examined at this time, you may see tiny white spots on the soft palate. These are called Koplik spots.

German measles is the infamous villain that produces birth defects when a pregnant woman contracts the disease. It is important, therefore, for women of childbearing age to know if they have had the disease and have thus been rendered immune to subsequent attacks. This information should be a part of the personal health record.

The onset of German measles may be heralded by a fever, feeling of illness, and swelling of lymph nodes behind the ears and at the base of the skull. The rash differs from measles in that after appearing on the face or chest, it spreads quickly over the body in a day or so. Old spots disappear as new ones turn up further down the body. The whole process takes only two or three days, while measles rash lasts at least a week.

If suspected, the presence of German measles should be confirmed by a doctor even if the ailment seems superficial. Then a positive record can be made for future reference.

Chicken pox, like the others, is preceded by illness and fever. While children usually get along with chicken pox tolerably well, adults may become severely ill. In any event, and in spite of its innocuous name, chicken pox should be seen by a doctor.

Red dots and then blisters appear on the trunk of the body. These blisters break and get crusty, and some may become pus-filled. Itching is likely to be severe. The illness will last a week or ten days and then the spots and sores will take somewhat longer to disappear.

Scarlet fever is a streptococcus infection which can lead to serious complications if left untreated; so a physician should always be consulted when it is suspected.

Scarlet fever is easy to confuse with measles at the outset, with the rash starting out as a redness about the neck and spreading to the rest of the body. The difference is that many dot-sized eruptions cover a bright red skin, making the skin feel rough. The face is flushed except for a rather obvious area around the mouth, which is a characteristic identifying mark of the disease. Peeling, similar to that caused by sunburn, occurs as the rash subsides.

NERVOUS, EMOTIONAL, OR PSYCHOLOGIC SKIN RESPONSES

One of the most mysterious and fascinating aspects of human skin is the way it is affected by the emotions, by stress or tension. When you consider how fear, joy, embarrassment, and other emotions are reflected in skin changes, it is not hard to believe that skin ailments may be affected by the emotions as well. It seems to be true, but it is still a facet of skin studies that is not at all understood by dermatologists.

We have seen how warts may appear to come and go at will or can be gotten rid of at times by psychic suggestion even though they are caused by a virus. The virus herpes simplex may inhabit skin cells for years and then suddenly cause a fever blister during a time of tension or upset. Flare-ups of acne, psoriasis, canker sores, and many other skin ailments have been seen to occur in patients under emotional stress. A rash, severe itching, or hives may occur with no better explanation than "nervousness" and may disappear mysteriously when the patient is told of the probably psychic cause of the ailment.

All this is not to say that a skin ailment should be ignored with the assumption, or the hope, that it is only "imagined" and will go away when one sets his thoughts straight. Far from it. Skin ailments should be seen by a professional and the source of the ailment should be scientifically established if at all possible. Then, the sufferer should be given emotional support and reassurance as well as medication, which is good therapy when dealing with any bodily ill.

CHAPTER 9

TESTS AND OBSERVATIONS OF THE REPRODUCTIVE ORGANS

Despite the deluge of revealing surveys and reports on human sexuality which have appeared during the past thirty years, it is still easier to find an honest politician than it is to find someone with an accurate knowledge of their reproductive organs. Most people have only the vaguest notion of how the reproductive systems work and just the sketchiest ideas of what equipment exists "down there," what it does, and what can go wrong.

Like other systems of the body, the reproductive systems are susceptible to a number of ailments. Unfortunately, the aura of mystery which surrounds the reproductive organs induces many people either to overestimate their problems or to turn a blind and embarrassed eye on signs of real trouble. This combination of misinformation and embarrassment exacts a high toll in death and disability, especially among women. Cancer of the breast, cervix, and uterus—where cure rates run better than 80 percent with early detection—together are the leading cause of death among women in their thirties and forties. And venereal disease continues as a major social scourge in spite of the availability of sure means to eradicate it and despite years of effort at public education.

The procedure for tracking the health of your reproductive system is the same as it is for the other body systems: you should know what organs are involved, where they are, and what they do; you should know what feels right and looks right for you when the system is functioning normally; and there are some basic tests and critical observations you should make to spot early signs of trouble, or to reassure yourself that all is going well.

THE FEMALE REPRODUCTIVE ORGANS

The External Genital Organs. The outer genital organs are collectively called the vulva, and this includes the whole area between the legs except for the anus. There is no reason why you can't examine this entire area if you want to, except that it takes a bit of arranging and a fair amount of flexibility. Most women feel that the lessons learned are well worth the effort, however. If you elect to try, you will need a medium-size mirror and a good light source to illuminate the area you are inspecting. Sit on the floor with your knees bent and spread apart, and arrange the mirror and light to get the best view possible. It's not an ideal way to do an examination, but it's the best you can do.

Beginning at the front, the most prominent feature is the mons, a pad of fatty tissue covering the pubic bone. This is the triangular area that is covered with pubic hair. The labia majora, the fleshy outer lips of the genitals, separate from the mons and proceed backward surrounding the outer organs and openings. Immediately below the mons is the clitoris, a tiny piece of very sensitive tissue, analogous in some ways to the male penis; it is largely made of erectile tissue, as the penis is, and both organs arise from the same site in a developing fetus. The difference is, of course, that the clitoris does not contain the urethra, the tube leading from the urinary bladder, and the penis does.

External Genital Organs of the Female

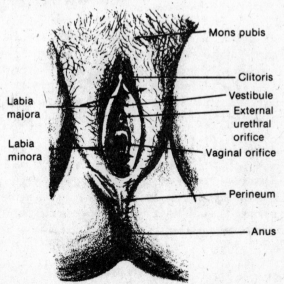

Mons pubis

Clitoris

Vestibule

External urethral orifice

Labia majora

Labia minora

Vaginal orifice

Perineum

Anus

The clitoris is partially hidden by the upper end of the labia minora, two thin folds of skin that follow along inside the labia majora. These form a hood over the clitoris in the front, and surround the urethral opening and the vaginal opening in an area called the vestibule. The urethra can be seen as a small protrusion just forward of the larger vaginal opening. You may also be able to see the hymen or its vestiges, a bit of membranous tissue that partially obstructs the lower end of the vagina. In a self-examination, this irregular fringe of tissue is sometimes mistaken for small growths, which it is not. The anus, the end of the digestive tract, is the obvious opening behind the vulva and is separated from it by an area known as the perineum.

The Internal Genital Organs.   The vagina is a thin-walled muscular tube whose lower opening we have just described in the vestibule of the vulva. It proceeds upward for about four inches until it meets the cervix, which is the opening into the uterus, or womb. The uterus is located just behind and above the bladder and in front of the rectum, which puts it just about in the middle of the body. If you draw a line around your body at about the level where bikini pants come, you will be pretty much in the plane of the uterus. Because a pregnancy shows somewhat higher than this, most people believe that the resting uterus is higher than it actually is.

Female Internal Reproductive Organs

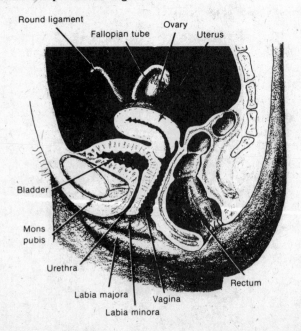

The uterus is not very large—only about the size of a small fist. The walls are relatively thick and muscular and the interior cavity is hardly more than a slit until it begins to expand to accommodate a growing fetus. Then the walls thicken and the internal cavity of the uterus expands dramatically. Extending outward from either side of the upper end of the uterus are the fallopian tubes, each of which is about four inches long. The ends of these tubes flare out, like the horn of a trumpet, and nestled in the shadow of each horn is an ovary about the size of a walnut.

The ovaries produce two female sex hormones, estrogen and progesterone, which encourage development of the female sex characteristics and regulate the menstrual cycle. In addition, each month one of the ovaries releases a mature egg. This is called ovulation. The egg is drawn into the horn-shaped end of the nearby fallopian tube where it makes its way to the uterus. If the egg is not fertilized along the way it disintegrates and is disposed of in vaginal secretions. Fertilization of a mature egg takes place in one of the fallopian tubes. When this happens the fertilized egg moves to the uterus where it becomes implanted in the uterine wall and begins to grow. When the fallopian tubes are blocked due to inflammation, scarring from disease, or for some other reason, fertilization can't take place and the woman is sterile. A sterilization procedure consists of tying off the fallopian tubes.

TROUBLE SIGNS IN THE EXTERNAL GENITAL ORGANS

The woman does not exist who has not had distress signals from her external genitals. These signals include unusual discharges, itching, burning, chafing, and pain in degrees ranging from petty annoyance to major discomfort. Sometimes lesions appear: sores, blisters, rashes, lumps, bumps, and so on.

No unusual sign or signal from the vulval region should be ignored if it persists more than a few days. You should not suffer stoically or embarrassedly waiting for itching or an abnormal discharge to "go away." Many rampaging and damaging infections can get a head start on you while you wait for them to cure themselves. A doctor should be consulted. As with any other complaint, the doctor will want as much information as you can give: the exact location of the problem, how it feels, how long you have been having trouble, and so on. You are best equipped to give this information when you know a bit about your anatomy and how it looks and feels under normal circumstances. In addition the doctor will want a good bit of history about your periods, any discharges you have noticed, what sort of life you lead, what sort of contraceptives you use, what douches, and even what sort of clothes you wear. And the more information you can provide from a personal health record, the more you will help the doctor to arrive at an exact diagnosis and precise treatment.

Self-diagnosis is difficult at best and impossible most of the time, but there are some observations you can make that will provide helpful information for your doctor. Following are some conditions that are definitely abnormal.

Contact or Allergic Vulvitis.   An -*itis* ending on a word means "inflammation of"—thus vulvitis means inflammation of the vulva, the external genitals.

This area can become inflamed as a result of direct contact with an irritating agent or as an allergic reaction to a substance taken internally. Women with sensitive skin may suffer a vulvar reaction as a result of contact with such seemingly innocent materials as perfumed toilet paper, bubble-bath products, douch ingredients, feminine spray deodorants, a new bath soap, or new synthetic fabrics in undergarments—especially in tight bikini pants. Similarly, vulvitis has also been diagnosed as an allergic reaction to common medications such as aspirin, sulfa drugs, and some laxatives.

Recognizing Contact or Allergic Vulvitis
This condition is indicated by a reddening of the vulvar skin accompanied by itching. In more severe cases the inner and outer vaginal lips may become swollen, and clear, bubblelike blisters may erupt; these will eventually drain and crust over.

Treatment consists of identifying the culprit and avoiding contact with it in the future. This is largely a trial and error process in which you identify recent changes regarding personal hygiene, such as a new girdle, the use of deodorized tampons or perfumed douches, contraceptive foams, or new medications including both over-the-counter and prescription drugs, and eliminating them one by one until you notice an improvement in your condition. Meanwhile, your doctor can prescribe soothing preparations to alleviate the more severe symptoms of contact or allergic vulvitis.

Genital Herpes.   Genital herpes is a disease caused by contact with the herpes simplex virus. There are actually two strains of this virus—the first, called herpes simplex type I, is responsible for the common cold sore and fever blister around the mouth and lips. A second, related strain, referred to as herpes simplex type II, affects the vulva, the upper vagina and the cervix. Recent studies indicate that either strain can be transmitted to the genitals, causing equally acute symptoms.

Recognizing Genital Herpes

Genital herpes is indicated by the presence of small, raised blisters along the vulva and the genital mucous membrane. In the course of a typical episode, which lasts from two to three weeks, the blisters develop into open sores with little holes in them; these become crusted, scabbed over, and finally, runny. This skin complaint can cause intense itching and distress and is usually accompanied by fever, swollen and painful lymph nodes in the groin area, and an overall rundown feeling. While the acute symptoms disappear when the infection has run its course, the virus continues to be harbored in the body and can flare up again without warning. Subsequent episodes of this recurring disease are usually milder than the initial attack.

As you can see, signs of genital herpes may be confused with the symptoms of severe contact or allergic vulvitis. If you have reason to believe you have contracted genital herpes, you should consult your doctor for a positive diagnosis and help in relieving its more distressing symptoms. Some doctors recommend a Pap smear every six months after genital herpes because of a suspected link with cervical cancer.

Enlarged Bartholin's Glands. Bartholin's glands are two small, mucous-producing glands located within the vestibule formed by the labia minora on either side of the vaginal opening. Normally you can neither see nor feel them. Occasionally, however, one or both of these glands can become blocked and subsequently infected, creating painful, pus-filled cysts.

Identifying Bartholin's Cysts

You can check for Bartholin's cysts by gently rolling the inner lips, or labia minora, on either side of the vaginal opening between your thumb and forefinger. A noticeable swelling that is tender to the touch is likely to be an enlarged Bartholin's gland and should be treated by your doctor. The pain, however, is likely to send you to the doctor before you bother to check yourself.

Genital Warts. Like warts elsewhere on the body, genital warts are caused by a virus. While they seem to be most commonly transmitted through sexual intercourse with an infected person, they can be acquired by other means as well.

Recognizing Genital Warts

In their early stages, genital warts are small, pinkish-tan growths not much bigger than a grain of rice. You may find two or three around the vaginal opening, or small clusters along the labia. They thrive on vaginal secretions, discharges, and moisture, and can be spread to other areas of the vulva by scratching. Once they have gained a foothold, genital warts can mushroom into large, cauliflowerlike masses. In extreme cases, they can interfere with intercourse, urination, and defecation.

KEEPING TRACK OF THE INTERNAL GENITAL ORGANS

Like other internal body organs, the internal genitals are best kept track of by observing how they function rather than by trying to examine them. Self-examination of the vagina and the cervix is possible, but it's rather too difficult for most people and the results are unreliable. However, if you are interested in trying a self-examination of these organs you can easily obtain an inexpensive vaginal speculum that is used to dilate the vagina, and you can find the procedure described in several recent books on popular gynecology.

But what is happening when all the organs of your reproductive system are working together is considerably more important than any single observation you may make with difficulty. As with other body systems you should observe what is normal for you and then be alert for changes that may signal all is not as it should be. Here are some things to watch for.

The Menstrual Cycle.   Menstrual periods should be regular and should not cause undue distress. Many women have a certain amount of pain with periods, but if you are regularly incapacitated when you are menstruating, this should be investigated by a gynecologist. If you have had relatively pain-free periods and suddenly have painful ones, you should seek medical advice; something may definitely be wrong.

Any change in the menstrual cycle is clearly an indication for a visit to the doctor. A number of disorders, both of the reproductive system and parts of the body nominally unrelated to the reproductive system, can affect the regularity of menstrual periods. For example, a change in the state of the thyroid gland almost always affects the menstrual cycle.

Vaginal Bleeding.   Unexpected vaginal bleeding is an important finding, and when this occurs, medical help should always be sought. Women who are taking birth control pills may have a phenomenon called breakthrough bleeding, which is slight bleeding or spotting between periods. This is generally nothing to be concerned about, but if it happens do two things: read the literature that comes with your birth control pills to see what it says about unexpected bleeding; then report the situation to your gynecologist to confirm that this is to be expected from your pill prescription.

An IUD may also cause unexpected bleeding and, once again, confirm with your doctor that this is normal. If you do not wear an IUD and you are not taking birth control pills, you should not bleed unless you are having a menstrual period. Other bleeding should be investigated professionally at once.

Pain.   Since all of the internal genital organs are located low in the pelvis, any problems related to these organs will generally center low in the torso, either in front or in back. But since this area also contains many other organs—the bladder, intestines, nerves, muscles, and so on—pain low in the torso is not indicative of any one thing; and if the pains don't persist they may be completely unimportant. But persistent pain anywhere in the body should be investigated.

Except for the first few times, intercourse should not cause pain. If intercourse becomes painful a physician should be consulted. Several diseases can cause painful intercourse and, as is true with male impotence, some psychological factors can cause painful intercourse as well. A woman should not assume that painful intercourse is a psychological problem, however, especially if she is happily married or has a satisfactory relationship with a man, without first consulting a gynecologist.

Vaginal Discharges.   Vaginal discharges are responsible for a wide range of complaints including itching, soreness and burning of the vulva, chafing of the inner thighs, and painful urination.

The mucous membranes that line the vagina secrete a small amount of milky discharge that lubricates the vagina just as saliva lubricates the mouth. Normally, these vaginal secretions have a slightly acidic pH value that kills yeast, fungi, and other harmful organisms. This delicate balance, however, can be upset by a number of factors including disease, an infection in some other part of the body, antibiotics, birth control pills, excessive douching, pregnancy, irritation of the vagina, a poor diet, or lack of sleep, to name just a few. When something happens to disturb the normal acidity of the vagina, other organisms normally held in check can multiply all out of proportion, resulting in an abnormal discharge that irritates the surrounding tissues.

Three of the most common offenders are *Trichomonas vaginalis*, better known as Trich or TV for short; *Candida albicana*, a fungal infection also called monilia or just yeast; and *Hemophilis vaginalis*, or HV, a bacterial infection. Diagnosing the exact culprit in a vaginal infection usually requires microscopic examination of the secretions, or a culture, and it is not uncommon to be afflicted by more than one infection at the same time. Generally you should be suspicious of any thick, copious, malodorous discharge that irritates or inflames the vagina or vulva. A good rule to apply to vaginal discharges is that they do not normally cause you discomfort. When they do, you should suspect a vaginal infection and see your doctor for treatment.

The Pap Smear.   A well-managed health-maintenance program for women must include an annual Pap smear. This is not an observation or test you can do yourself, but it is worth discussing for a moment because of its importance as a lifesaving technique and because certain misconceptions about what it does seem to persist in spite of two decades of publicity and education by various health agencies.

Cervical and uterine cancers are the third leading cause of death among women in some age groups. It is an important killer in all age groups, even among women in their twenties. When discovered early, however, cure rates for cervical and uterine cancers are extremely high. The purpose of the Pap smear is to make early discovery of the presence of cancer cells in the uterus.

Keep in mind that the Pap smear is only a cancer test; it doesn't test for venereal disease or pregnancy or monilia or anything else. The test is named for Dr. Papanicalou who invented the staining technique that is needed to study the sample cells under a microscope. Most doctors routinely do the test as part of a gynecological examination.

A speculum is inserted into the vagina to expand the canal and permit examination of the vaginal walls and the cervix. The doctor then gently scrapes a few loose surface cells from the cervix with a small wooden or plastic paddle. These cells are immediately smeared on a microscope slide and sprayed with a special fixative. The fixed slide is then sent to a medical laboratory where it is stained to make microscopic examination of the cells possible.

The slides are interpreted as being one of six groups: Class 0 means the sample is inadequate for diagnosis for some reason; Class 1 means that the cells are entirely normal; Class 2 is negative for cancer but the technician has found some other kinds of abnormal cells that should be looked into; Class 3 means that cancer cells are suspected; Class 4 is positive for cancer; and Class 5 is strongly positive for cancer. Your doctor will let you know if your test is other than Class 1.

Testing for Ovulation.   As we pointed out earlier, a single mature egg erupts from one of the ovaries once a month, is caught in the hornlike end of a fallopian tube and makes its way to the uterus. If the egg is fertilized on the way, a pregnancy begins. If the egg is not fertilized by a male sperm within about twelve hours, the egg disintegrates and is disposed of. Thus a woman is fertile for a very short period every month.

The eruption of an egg from an ovary is called ovulation, and it occurs about fourteen days from the *beginning* of a menstrual period. Being able to identify the time of ovulation can serve two purposes: If you want to become pregnant, this is the best time for intercourse. If you do not want to become pregnant and you are not using other contraceptive methods, you will want to abstain from intercourse four or five days before you ovulate and a couple of days afterward. This is the basis of the rhythm method of contraception. Since the egg released by the ovary has an active life of about twelve hours and male sperm can survive two or three days after intercourse, if you wish to minimize your chances of becoming pregnant you can calculate when *not* to have intercourse. What makes the rhythm method unreliable is that menstrual cycles are not always precisely on schedule and this often throws off the calculations just enough to allow fertilization to occur.

You can identify the time of your ovulation, however, by tracking your basal body temperature. Your basal body temperature (BBT) is the temperature of your body at complete rest. This temperature is taken orally immediately upon awakening in the morning and is usually about one and one-half degrees lower than your normal body temperature. If you were to take your BBT each morning, you would notice a slight drop immediately followed by a sharp rise in temperature approximately two weeks from the first day of your menstrual period. This monthly rise in the BBT is triggered by ovulation, which stimulates hormone production. By charting your basal body temperature over a period of months, you can determine when you are ovulating and identify the short period of fertility. It will also show if, indeed, you *are* ovulating, which is the first thing a doctor will want to know if you are having trouble becoming pregnant when you want to.

Checking Ovulation by Tracking Basal Body Temperature

You will need a basal body temperature thermometer. This is a special oral thermometer with a scale of 95-100°F. with widely spaced, tenth-degree gradations that make it easy for you to detect slight variations in temperature. An ordinary fever thermometer will work, but will not be as easy to read.

1. Using a sheet of graph paper, prepare a chart of your menstrual cycle.

Across the top of the chart, list the days in your menstrual cycle. The first day of your menstrual period is day #1. If your cycle is normally 28 days long, your chart will be 28 squares across. If your period comes every 31 days, your chart will be 31 squares across, and so on. Down the left-hand side of the chart, mark degrees in temperature, from 99.0°F. down to 96.5 or lower in tenth-degree gradations.

2. Beginning with the first day of your menstrual flow, start tracking your basal body temperature. Keep your thermometer on your bedside table and pop it into your mouth first thing in the morning *before* you get out of bed or before you are even fully awake. Be sure it has been properly shaken down the night before so it is ready to use. Record your temperature each day by locating the temperature registered on your thermometer in the left-hand column of your chart, and then follow this line across until you come to the square under the appropriate day of your cycle. Make a little *x* at this spot.

3. At the end of your cycle, draw a line connecting the *x*'s you have charted. Repeat this procedure for three to four months. You now have a graphic depiction of your ovulatory cycle.

If you are ovulating, you will notice a drop immediately followed by a sharp rise of between .5 and 1.0° in your basal body temperature. This will happen around the fourteenth day of each cycle. The low point represents the time of ovulation. When your temperature goes back up it will stay there, with slight variations, until two or three days prior to the onset of your next menstrual period, at which point your BBT drops and a new cycle begins. If you fail to ovulate in any given cycle, your BBT will not vary by more than two or three tenths of a degree for the whole cycle. If, on the other hand, you ovulate and the egg is fertilized, your

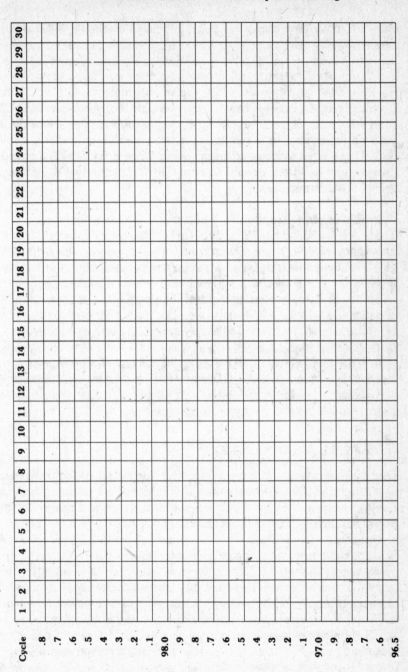

BASAL BODY TEMPERATURE CHART

Cycle	1	2	3	4	5	6	7	8	9	10	11	12	13	14	15	16	17	18	19	20	21	22	23	24	25	26	27	28	29	30
.8																														
.7																														
.6																														
.5																														
.4																														
.3																														
.2																														
.1																														
98.0																														
.9																														
.8																														
.7																														
.6																														
.5																														
.4																														
.3																														
.2																														
.1																														
97.0																														
.9																														
.8																														
.7																														
.6																														
96.5																														

BBT will remain elevated. This is one of the earliest signs of a possible pregnancy.

Pregnancy Testing.   Of all the medical tests for women, pregnancy testing is surely near the top of the most wanted list. Until recently, women had to leave a urine sample with their doctor, who then forwarded it to a medical laboratory for testing. Now do-it-yourself pregnancy testing kits are available in drugstores for about $10. These offer obvious advantages including privacy and a speedy diagnosis. When used according to the instructions, they are purportedly 97 percent accurate.

Do-It-Yourself Pregnancy Testing

There are a number of kits on the market that allow you to verify a pregnancy in the privacy of your own home as early as the ninth day after the day you expected your period to begin. All of them check for the presence of a special pregnancy hormone in the urine.

Such kits typically consist of a test tube containing special reagent chemicals, a vial of purified water, a dropper with a squeeze bulb, and a test-tube holder. The test is relatively simple to perform and involves placing a few drops of a first-morning urine sample in the test tube, adding the purified water, and shaking vigorously. Then you place the test tube in its special holder, let it stand undisturbed for two hours, and then read the results. A dark brown, donut-shaped ring in the test-tube solution indicates a positive test for pregnancy.

BREAST SELF-EXAMINATION

One of the most widely recognized tests for detecting cancer in women is self-examination of the breasts. This involves a monthly examination in which you observe and feel for characteristic changes in the breast indicating the presence of a growth which was not there before.

Many women mistakenly assume that a test they can do themselves is probably inferior to a doctor's examination. Actually, quite the opposite is true in this case. If you examine your breasts thoroughly and faithfully each month, you are in a much better position to detect small changes than your doctor, who only does an examination once a year. In fact, many more breast cancers are discovered by women themselves than by any physician or sophisticated breast-cancer detection method. If caught early, the chances are excellent you can be completely cured of the disease. The key element is time—the longer a cancer has to grow and spread to other parts of the body, the harder it is to cure. Thus any suspicious changes you may discover in your monthly examination should be treated as a medical emergency. While most lumps in the breast turn out to be benign—that is, noncancerous—a lump should always be assumed cancerous until proven otherwise by your doctor.

A word or two here about the anatomy of the breast may help you to better understand what you will see and feel in your self-examination. The breasts contain a substantial amount of fat. Large breasts contain more fat than smaller breasts. This fat is interspersed with fine, ligamentous structures which give the breast its shape and prevent it from sagging. In older women, this ligamentous structure becomes somewhat stretched so that the breasts have a tendency to sag a bit. The breasts also contain alveolar glands, each with its own duct called a lactiferous duct. The glands produce milk when a baby is born, and the ducts transport the milk to the surface in the center of the nipple area.

In the nonlactating breast—that is, a breast which is not producing milk—the milk glands are small, pea-sized structures distributed more or less randomly around the central area of the breast. You may be able to feel some of them. Because the milk glands are buried in the fat structure, you will not feel them on the surface of the breast tissue but,

The Breast

rather, deep inside. They are not particularly tender to the touch and their size does not vary significantly from month to month.

It is easy at first to mistake the milk glands for tumors, and it is a fact that most breast tumors do grow either in the milk glands themselves or in the duct structures. But as you become familiar with your own breasts, you will know which milk glands can be felt; consequently, you will be able to recognize an abnormal lump that wasn't there before.

All women should examine their breasts on a regular monthly basis. This is best done about one week after the end of the menstrual period. At this time, the breasts are usually neither tender nor swollen. The swelling and tenderness of the breasts which often accompany the menstrual period are caused by cyclic hormonal changes. After menopause, these changes no longer occur and breast self-examination should be carried out on a regular calendar basis, such as the first of each month. If a woman is no longer having menstrual periods because of a hysterectomy, she should check with her doctor about the best time to perform breast self-examination. If she is still relatively young and the hysterectomy did not involve both ovaries, her body will still be undergoing cyclic hormonal changes and the breasts should not be examined during the swollen, tender period. If both ovaries have been removed, she will likely be receiving some kind of hormone therapy and instructions about breast self-examination should be sought from the doctor.

Breast Self-Examination

This test should be performed with the hand flat and the fingers together. Do not approach the examination timidly with the tips of one or two fingers, or by pinching bits of tissue between the thumb and forefinger. The examination will be much more successful if all four fingers, flattened together, are used.

1. The first step of the examination should be carried out during a shower or bath when your hands can glide easily over the wet, soapy skin. With your fingers flat, move your hand gently over every part of the breast and check for any lumps, hard knots, or thickening. Use the right hand to examine the left breast and the left hand to examine the right breast. Do not limit your examination to just the central part of the breast. Cover the entire area from the middle of your chest to the middle of the side of your body, including the armpits. Also be sure you examine both high enough and low enough.

Get to know your breasts. If in the first examination you discover one or two particular milk glands, try to identify them again another day. It is very unlikely that you will find a tumor on the first examination; the success of the technique depends upon each woman learning the normal anatomy of her own breasts and then perhaps some day discovering that something new has appeared and that there has been a change in the normal anatomy.

2. The second step consists of critical observation. Stand in front of a mirror and inspect your breasts with your arms at your sides. Both breasts will not appear to be the same. One will probably hang a little lower than the other, and one may be a trifle larger than the other. Few women have breasts which, on careful examination, are identical.

Observe the contour of your breasts. Look for any swelling, lumps, dimpling of the skin, or any changes in the nipples. These are all important. After observing your breasts with your arms at your sides, raise your arms straight up over your head and hold them high. This lifts the breasts up and changes their shape a bit. Again, look at the shape and contour of each breast for indications of swelling, dimpling of the skin, or changes in the nipple. You may see some changes with your arms held high over your head which are not apparent when your arms are at your sides. Finally, rest the palms of your hands on your hips and press down firmly. This tightens your chest muscles and further modifies the contour and shape of the breasts. Again, look for swelling, lumps, dimpling of the skin, and changes in the nipple.

Skin changes and dimpling of the skin are just as significant as lumps. As explained earlier, the breasts contain many small, ligamentous structures, and a small tumor growing along one of the milk ducts may slightly displace one of these ligaments. The small amount of tension placed on the ligament by the tumor will show itself on the surface as a dimple, even though the tumor itself is not large enough to show on the surface as a lump or swelling. Dimpling and skin changes are therefore very important findings.

Any change in the nipple is important for the same reason. The nipple normally sticks out. A small tumor, however, may press on one or two of the milk ducts in such a way that the milk ducts pull the nipple in toward the breast. Thus if a nipple becomes abnormally inverted, this is probably significant.

3. The third step in your examination of the breasts is carried out lying down. Lie down on your bed comfortably on your back. Once again you will be examining your right breast with your left hand and your left breast with your right hand.

Start with the right breast. Place a pillow or fold a towel under your right shoulder and put your right hand behind your head. This position tends to make the breast spread out a bit and distributes the breast tissue more evenly over the chest wall. With the fingers of the left hand held flat, press gently around the breast in clockwise motion. Starting at the top of your breast where twelve o'clock might be on a clock face, move around the clock until you have made a full circle back to twelve. A ridge of firm tissue in the lower curve is perfectly normal. Be sure you follow the outer edge of the breast far enough out toward the armpit. When you have made the first complete circle, move about one inch in toward the nipple and start another circle at twelve o'clock. Continue making concentric circles until you have examined every part of your breast including the nipple. This generally requires four or five circles. Since you are looking for relatively small lumps, be sure not to make the space between the circles too large. Also, do not ignore the nipples. Breast tumors can occur in any area of the breast, including directly under the nipple structure.

When you have finished examining the right breast, place the towel or pillow under your left shoulder, put your left hand behind your head, and examine your left breast with your right hand, repeating the procedure described above.

In this step of the examination you will be looking mostly for lumps. You will always find plenty of lumps which are the normal gland tissue within the breast. After a few examinations you will learn to recognize these gland structures and you will begin to know the location of many of the glands in both your breasts. Some women's breasts are normally much lumpier than others, so don't be alarmed if you find a great many lumps in your breasts and a friend reports finding very few in hers.

Finally, squeeze each nipple gently between the thumb and index finger. Normally, nothing should come out. Any discharge, either clear or bloody, should be reported to your doctor.

Once you have been examining your breasts on a regular basis, any abnormality which you find is most likely to start out as something quite small and this is when you want to discover it. Don't expect a lump the size of a golf ball or even a cherry to suddenly show up. You are much more likely to find something the size of an orange seed or smaller which you haven't noticed before. Pay attention to the consistency of the little lumps which are your normal milk glands. If you find something suspicious, it is likely to have a consistency somewhat different, often harder, than that of your normal gland structures. However, consistency is not an infallible indicator of a tumor and you should be much more concerned with finding a small lump in a location where you are quite certain no lumps existed the previous month. Remember, you are primarily looking for changes.

FOR YOUR PERSONAL HEALTH RECORD

   1. Describe a typical menstrual period you consider usual and normal—

     a. Cycle: number of days; regular, irregular.
     b. Describe the extent of any discomfort.
     c. Light or heavy flow; duration.

   2. Describe any distress or copious discharge you notice occurring in the vulvar area regularly or persistently.
   3. Record the date of your last Pap smear.
   4. Record the date of each breast self-examination.

VENEREAL DISEASE

So much has been said about syphilis and gonorrhea ever since the fruitless campaigns to eliminate them among soldiers and sailors in World War II, that any further descriptions of them would seem superfluous. But despite the most widespread educational programs ever launched against specific diseases, and despite easy availability of certain cure for all who seek it, syphilis and gonorrhea continue to hold their own as cripplers and killers in our society. So another word or two about venereal disease is probably in order.

   Gonorrhea.   Gonorrhea is second only to the common cold as the most prevalent communicable disease in the United States. Unlike the common cold, however, most women infected with gonorrhea don't even know they have it. In fact, 80 percent will be completely asymptomatic—that is, free of overt symptoms which would alert them to the presence of this venereal disease. But as the bacteria which causes gonorrhea works its way up the vagina, through the cervix and into the uterus, the disease can spread to the fallopian tubes, resulting in scarring of the tubes and permanent sterility.

   Early symptoms of gonorrhea in women, when they occur, include burning and frequent urination, which may be mistaken for a passing bladder infection, and a thick greenish-yellow discharge which is almost impossible to distinguish from nonvenereal discharges without a culture test. A culture test involves smearing a sample of the discharge on a special culture plate that encourages the growth of the gonococcus bacteria, incubating it for a period of time, and then examining the culture for characteristic signs indicating the presence of *Neisseria gonorrhoeae*.

Traditionally, this test has been done almost exclusively in medical laboratories by technicians who prepare a culture and interpret the results of specimens sent to them by doctors. In recent years, however, medical manufacturers have developed a diagnostic test for gonorrhea that can be performed by a doctor or informed assistant in the doctor's office and does not have to be sent out to a laboratory. One such test developed by Smith-Kline is called the Isocult™ Diagnostic Culturing System. This is essentially a self-contained culture kit in a test tube. Its basic components are a paddle impregnated with a special culture medium onto which you apply the specimen to be tested, a test tube into which the paddle is inserted, and a compact, desk-top incubator which provides the proper temperature for incubating the culture. The Isocult™ system offers nine different tests, including tests for two vaginal infections and strep throat as well as the test for gonorrhea. The price per test is reasonable—about $5 per test plus approximately $30 for the incubating unit—and it can be performed by anyone who can follow directions intelligently. At the present time these kits are not available to the public for home use. With medical self-help becoming more and more popular, however, it is highly possible that such kits will become available at the corner drugstore along with the currently popular urine and pregnancy tests.

Syphilis.   While gonorrhea is the second leading reported communicable disease in this country, syphilis is not far behind, ranking third. The confirming test for syphilis is a blood test which must be done by a doctor or medical laboratory. If you suspect you may have been exposed to syphilis and you can't or don't want to contact a local doctor, call your state department of health, the United States Public Health Service, or walk into any hospital with an emergency receiving division and explain your problem.

Even the vaguest suspicion that a sexual partner may have been infected should be enough to cause you to have a blood test. And a suspicion is all you may have until symptoms become manifest, because infectious syphilis in a partner is rarely obvious. Then, your own symptoms may come and go with minimum discomfort so that you can be lulled into complacency until it is too late for successful treatment.

Signs and Symptoms of Syphilis

If you have been exposed to syphilis within the last nine to ninety days, your examination of the vulva may reveal a single, painless sore known as a chancre. This represents the site where the corkscrew-shaped spirochete that causes syphilis entered your body. The chancre is painless, round, slightly raised, and has a hard base that may feel as if there is a nickel or a dime buried under the skin. A syphilitic chancre is commonly accompanied by painless, hard, swollen lymph nodes in the area of the groin. If the chancre is hidden within the vaginal canal, you may miss it in a casual examination.

While the spirochete may penetrate any skin area or mucous membrane—such as the lips, tongue, and tonsils—its most common site of entry is the genital area. You should thoroughly inspect the inner and outer lips of the vagina for this characteristic sore. Left alone, the chancre will heal in thirty to ninety days, but the spirochetes remain and continue to multiply and circulate in the bloodstream. The secondary stage of syphilis is indicated by a generalized skin rash which appears anywhere from a few days to a few weeks after the chancre heals. (For a more detailed description of the rash of secondary syphilis, see the chapter on the skin.)

MALE REPRODUCTIVE ORGANS

Unlike the female, who must go to some lengths just to view the outer fringes of her reproductive system, the male can easily examine his primary sexual organs—the penis and the two testicles contained in the scrotum. The path of the sperm from the testicles to the penis, however, is by no means as direct as many men imagine. Along the way are a number of related organs and glands located within the body cavity and connected by a considerable amount of plumbing in the form of ducts and tubes.

The sperm which ultimately fertilize the female egg is manufactured in the two testicles. These are contained in a small sac called the scrotum which hangs outside the main body cavity, just behind and below the penis. This arrangement provides precise temperature control for the production of healthy sperm by allowing the testicles to draw close to the body for warmth or drop down to cool off. From the tubules where they are manufactured, the sperm move into the

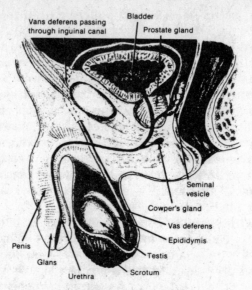

The Male Reproductive Organs

epididymis, a sort of holding area within the scrotum which curves over the back and top of each testicle. Here, the immature sperm can mature before continuing on to the vasa deferentia (singular: vas deferens).

The vasa deferentia are the two ducts which conduct the sperm out of the testicles and up into the main body cavity. These slender ducts circle around the bladder, enlarge just a bit to form the ampulla, and then narrow into the ejaculatory ducts which pierce the back of the prostate. The prostate is a gland about the size of a walnut which is situated at the neck of the bladder and surrounds the urethra, through which urine passes. Directly below the ampulla, which is the expanded portion of the vas deferens, is a pouchlike structure called the seminal vesicle. This gland makes and secretes fluid which feeds into the ejaculatory duct, where it mixes with sperm from the ampullar portion of the vas.

Up to this point, the male reproductive organs have been paired—two testicles, two epididymides, two vasa deferentia, two ampullae, two seminal vesicles, two ejaculatory ducts. But at the site of the prostate everything leaves through one tube—the urethra. The urethra exits to the outside through the penis, which is an erectile organ composed chiefly of spongelike tissue. When sexually aroused, this spongelike tissue becomes engorged with blood, causing the penis to become firm and erect. During ejaculation, the ejaculatory ducts empty into the urethra, the prostate gland contributes some fluids of its own, and the mixture, called semen, is forced out the urethra by muscular contractions. At the same time, a circular muscle around the neck of the bladder closes tightly to prevent urine from passing into the urethra or semen from backing up into the bladder.

To many men the whole process is nothing short of miraculous, and the fear that something might threaten its continued functioning is never far from their minds. Usually, such fears are greatly exaggerated. But it's a good idea nevertheless to keep a weather-eye on this vital area by periodically performing the following tests, checks, and examinations.

Checking the Scrotum, Testicles, and the Inguinal Crease. A good place to begin is the scrotum. First, check to see that both testicles have descended into the scrotal sac; it is not uncommon for young boys, or adults for that matter, to have an undescended testicle. This condition should be seen by a doctor.

Compare the relative size of the two testicles—they should be approximately equal, each being about the size of a small plum. The left testicle normally hangs a bit lower than the right. Gently palpate both testicles and note if there is any extreme sensitivity. Now examine the entire scrotum for lumps. Virtually any kind of a lump or mass which appears within the scrotum is abnormal. Small, relatively hard lumps which suddenly appear within the scrotum may be the first sign of a malignant tumor and medical attention should be sought immediately.

Small lumps which appear in the inguinal area—that is, in the crease where the legs join the body—are likely to be swollen lymph nodes. These nodes can swell for a variety of reasons which often have nothing to do with the genitals. For example, an infection in a leg or foot can cause swelling of the lymph nodes in the inguinal area on that side of the body. If these persist, they should be shown to a doctor.

Hernia. A soft mass within or just above the scrotum may be due to an inguinal hernia. A hernia is a portion of tissue or part of an organ that has protruded through a weakness or abnormal opening in any part of the body. One of the most common hernias, called an inguinal hernia, involves a loop of bowel that has worked its way into the inguinal canal.

Up until a month or so before birth, the testicles of the male fetus are situated in the abdomen. The inguinal canals are the natural passages through which they descend into the scrotum. This happens shortly before or shortly after birth, whereupon the passages close. Occasionally, however, the inguinal canals do not close completely and remain as weak spots in the abdominal wall. Any strain causing increased abdominal pressure—such as heavy lifting, violent games, chronic cough, or constipation—can accentuate this weakness and eventually reopen a canal. As continued pressure increases the size of the opening, a loop of bowel can work its way into the passage and eventually enter the scrotum. While this condition can take many years of straining and pushing to develop, inguinal hernias are as common in boys as in grown men.

A hernia is a serious finding because of the possibility that the loop of bowel may become twisted, cutting off the supply of blood to that portion of tissue. This is called a strangulated hernia and necessitates emergency surgery to prevent a serious gangrenous condition from setting in.

Testing for Hernia

A soft mass in the scrotum or in the area just above either testicle may be an inguinal hernia.

One test you can do which indicates a hernia condition is to try to "reduce" the mass by manipulating the loop of bowel so that it slides back up into the abdominal cavity. Lie down on your back with your feet elevated and gently manipulate the mass with your fingers. Generally, an inguinal hernia can be maneuvered back into the abdomen. If this is not possible, the mass may be a hydrocele (see below) instead of a hernia.

A second test you can make to check for hernia is the cough test. Stand in front of a full-length mirror, naked, so that you have a good view of the genital area. Now, cough hard and strain in the abdominal area. As you do this, watch the groin area just above the scrotum for a bulge that was not apparent before, or ask someone to watch closely for you. Any bulge in the area of the groin that is induced by coughing should be checked out by your doctor.

Hydrocele.   A soft mass in the scrotum may also indicate a hydrocele. A hydrocele is a cystic accumulation of fluid within a little sac which forms above the testicle in the scrotum. While this is not a dangerous condition, it can cause considerable discomfort and should be brought to the attention of your physician.

Transillumination Test for a Hydrocele

You can test to determine if a mass in the scrotum is a hydrocele using an ordinary flashlight. Switch the flashlight on and press it up tight against the back side of the scrotum. If the mass lights up and glows like a dull, red-orange light bulb, it is most likely a hydrocele. If, however, light is not transmitted through the mass, it is more likely to be a hernia or some other growth.

Varicocele.   Each of the testicles in the scrotum is suspended by a cordlike structure consisting of the vas deferens, through which sperm passes, and a number of veins, arteries, lymphatic vessels, and nerves. This structure is called the spermatic cord and the veins that contribute to it are referred to as the testicular veins. These testicular veins can become varicose—that is, enlarged and dilated. This condition is known as a varicocele and occurs almost exclusively in the left spermatic cord.

Checking for a Varicocele

The presence of a varicocele is indicated by a swelling in the upper scrotum coupled with an abnormal tenderness of the spermatic cord on that side. To check for this condition, locate the spermatic cords on each side of the scrotum. You can easily feel this structure about midway between the testicle and the point at which the scrotum joins the body. Gently palpate the cord between your thumb and forefinger. A light touch here should not cause undue discomfort. If, however, you perceive a noticeable swelling that is painful to the touch, you should have your physician examine the cord for a possible varicocele.

Recognizing Prostate Trouble.   The prostate gland contributes some important nutrients to the seminal fluid that provide nourishment for the sperm as they swim up the female vaginal tract toward the egg. Its design, however, is generally counted as one of nature's engineering nightmares. The prostate is located at the base of the bladder, where it surrounds the urethra like a donut. When this gland enlarges, as it frequently does, it can effectively slow and eventually shut off the flow of urine from the bladder. If left untreated, severe discomfort and eventual damage to the bladder and kidneys can result.

It has been estimated that at least 50 percent of all men over the age of fifty are likely to develop some form of prostate trouble, and the risk accelerates with advancing age. Prostate disorders fall into three categories: Infectious prostatitis is an inflammation of the prostate gland caused by a bacterial or a viral infection; the *Escherichia coli* bacilli found in the lower bowel and feces and the gonococcus bacilli are two common offenders here. Benign prostatic hypertrophy, or simply BPH, is an enlargement of the prostate gland which is not cancerous. Prostate cancer, a malignant enlargment of the prostate, is a much rarer condition than simple hypertrophy.

Due to its location within the body, you cannot perform an effective self-examination of the prostate. A doctor will check the prostate by inserting a gloved finger into the rectum and palpating the gland through the rectal wall to feel for lumps, swellings, or tenderness. Even if you could duplicate this procedure, it is unlikely that you would have sufficient expertise to interpret what you feel. There are, however, some signs and symptoms you can observe that are indicative of prostate trouble. Some of the more common are:

- Frequent, urgent, and painful or difficult urination which may cause you to get up to go to the bathroom two, three or more times a night.
- Difficulty in beginning to urinate.
- A feeling that the bladder has not been emptied completely.
- Blood in the urine.
- A burning sensation in the urethra upon urination or after ejaculation.
- Pain in the lower back or the perineal area (the area between the anus and the scrotum).

Some of these symptoms, of course, could be caused by problems other than disorders of the prostate, such as bladder infections. In any case, you should report such warning signs promptly and accurately to your doctor for a professional evaluation.

Many of the afflictions discussed in connection with the female genitals apply to the male genitals also.

Genital Warts.   As in the female, genital warts in the male thrive on moisture. Thus penile discharges, sweat, and other secretions provide them with an environment that must seem made-to-order. Look for small clusters of pinkish-tan growths not much larger than a grain of rice on the penis, the scrotum, and around the anus. They begin small, but can dramatically mushroom into large, cauliflowerlike masses. Scratching can spread the infection and sexual intercourse can pass it on to your partner.

Genital Herpes.   This also follows a similar course in men and women. The first sign is likely to be several small, red bumps on the penis which generally appear two to eight days after intercourse with an infected person. These bumps quickly escalate into tiny, painful blisters filled with a clear fluid. As white blood cells move into the blisters to combat the virus, this fluid becomes cloudy. At this stage the blisters rupture, leaving small, wet open sores that are still painful and still infectious. About ten days after their first appearance, the sores crust over, pain gradually subsides, and healing follows. The entire episode is often accompanied by fever, swollen lymph glands in the groin, and burning on urination. A relapse may strike about six to eight weeks later, and subsequent episodes can recur periodically throughout life, though these are usually less severe than the initial bout.

Syphilis. Detecting primary syphilis in men, as in women, involves finding its characteristic sore, called a chancre, on the genitals, mouth, or anus. The chancre is painless, round, slightly raised, and has a hard base that may feel as if there is a coin embedded in the skin. It lasts about two to six weeks and then heals by itself, even without treatment. Long before this, however, the spirochete that causes syphilis has entered the bloodstream.

Syphilis may be detected during its secondary stage by a generalized skin rash which appears anywhere from a few days to a few weeks after the chancre heals. Either of these symptoms, or merely the suspicion that you have been exposed to syphilis, should prompt a visit to your doctor for a confirmed diagnosis and treatment. (A more detailed description of the rash of secondary syphilis is included in the chapter dealing with skin problems.)

Gonorrhea. Whereas gonorrhea in women often goes unnoticed at first, a gonorrheal infection in men usually announces its presence within a week after exposure with two unmistakable symptoms which often encourage a man to go to the doctor. The first is a discharge of pus from the opening of the penis, and the second is a burning sensation when passing urine. Other infections, some sexually acquired and some not, can cause the same symptoms. In any case, they should be seen by a doctor.

As mentioned earlier, simple culture tests for gonorrhea exist and may one day join other self-diagnosis kits, such as pregnancy and urine testing, on drugstore shelves.

CHAPTER 10

TRACKING AND TESTING THE HEALTH AND DEVELOPMENT OF CHILDREN

Babies and children are in a continual state of change. Seemingly overnight, they acquire new skills and new interests. They outgrow toys they played with yesterday and clothes they wore last week. Before you have even ceased marveling at their latest triumph, they surprise you with a new word, a new accomplishment, an unexpected talent, a new insight.

But despite their infinite variety, children are pretty predictable in many ways. People who have observed large numbers of children from infancy through adolescence have noticed that, by and large, most babies tend to walk at an average age, use a few words at about the same time, and demonstrate improved coordination from year to year. Similarly, older children generally grow at predictable rates and mature physically at an age consistent with their previous growth pattern.

You will probably never totally fathom your child's unique personality, but you can keep a watchful eye on your child's health and development by keeping a record of growth and monitoring motor and perceptual progress. In this way, you will be in a good position to spot any abnormality and bring it to the attention of your pediatrician. And almost invariably, the earlier a problem is spotted, the better it responds to treatment.

While many of the tests and observations described earlier in this book are equally applicable to children and adults, the material that follows should give you some additional insights into the special problems and characteristics of infants and children.

GROWTH

One of the most common concerns voiced by parents is whether or not a child is growing normally. In order to assess a child's rate of growth, it is necessary to understand what is meant by the terms "normal" and "average."

Some people are short and some people are tall; some people mature quickly while others mature more slowly. This is a normal phenomenon. An adult who is 6 feet 6 inches tall is just as normal as one who is 5 feet tall. There is an 18-inch difference in height, but neither person is tagged as being abnormal because of this difference. Similarly, some children seem to develop and mature more rapidly while others go through the same process but require a little more time. Neither the rapidly developing child nor the slowly developing child is considered abnormal as long as the development stays within a range of normal variability. This variability in heights and weights and rates of development can be shown on what statisticians call a "normal distribution curve."

If one measures a large number of people and then makes a graph showing the number of people found to be 5 feet tall, and then the number found to be 5 feet 1 inch, 5 feet 2 inches, and so forth, all the way up to 6 feet 6 inches tall, one would find that there are relatively few people who are less than 5 feet tall and also relatively few who are more than 6 feet 6 inches tall. Somewhere in the middle of this range, about 5 feet 6 inches or 5 feet 7 inches, one finds the greatest number of people. The numbers diminish as the heights get shorter and the numbers also diminish as the heights get taller. This curve or plot of the numbers of people of any given height is the normal distribution curve. The curve vaguely resembles the silhouette of a bell and is therefore sometimes referred to as a bell curve.

What this curve tells us is that there are more persons of middle height than there are short ones or tall ones. Similarly, in other categories, there are more middle-weight people than there are light ones or heavy ones, and there are more middle-intelligence people than there are super bright or unusually dull ones. The people represented by the center or highest point of the curve are the "average" people.

From the above discussion it should be clear that a large number of people are indeed average in many respects. There are also, however, large numbers of people whose height or weight or whatever you are measuring falls at either one end of the curve or the other. These people are clearly not average, because they are taller or shorter or heavier or lighter than those who fall in the middle of the curve; but they are still normal and simply fall either at one end or the other of the normal distribution curve.

It is therefore impossible to say that a specific height or a specific weight is normal for a child at any given age. Heights and weights and other growth statistics must always be expressed in "ranges of normal." The average eight-year-old boy weighs 55 pounds, but an eight-year-old boy who weighs only 48 pounds is certainly not abnormal. Both boys are probably entirely normal but one simply weighs a bit less than the other. In fact, the normal weight for eight-year-old boys ranges from about 45 to 77 pounds. Though most boys fall in the middle of this range, those at either end are just as normal as those in the middle.

Obviously, not every individual's growth is normal, and a line has to be drawn somewhere to differentiate between growth rates that are normal and those that are not. In considering this distinction, statisticians have found that those who fall in the lowest 3 to 5 percent on the graph and those who fall in the highest 3 to 5 percent are most likely to be abnormal. Therefore, normal has been defined as all those individuals who fall within the normal distribution curve *except* those who are in the bottom and the top 5 percent.

Tracking Your Child's Growth.   Keeping track of your child's growth rate is important because it can alert you to a significant deviation in the child's expected pattern of growth. For instance, a child who has been growing steadily at an average rate can be expected to continue at about the same pace. A sudden falling off in the normal growth rate or a standstill in growth should be investigated.

You should start tracking your child's growth from infancy by measuring length, weight, and head circumference on a monthly basis.

How to Measure an Infant

1. *Length.* Length may be the most difficult measurement in an infant simply because babies tend to squirm a bit. The infant should be lying flat on its back with the soles of the feet braced up against a board. Place the lower end of a yardstick against the board and, making sure that the baby's legs are fully extended, locate the top of the baby's head along the measuring stick and read the length. After about eighteen months some babies will be more than three feet long, so a tape measure or other device longer than a yardstick will be required. At about two and a half years of age, or whenever the child can stand erect, length can be measured in the standard manner.

2. *Weight.* Infants can be weighed using either a baby scale or a conventional bathroom scale. To use the latter, weigh yourself first and

record the weight, then weigh yourself holding the infant or young child. The additional pounds are what the baby weighs. Bathroom scales, of course, are only accurate to the nearest pound.

3. *Head circumference.* The head circumference is taken with a tape measure drawn snugly around the skull at its maximum diameter. The tape should be about level with the eyebrows in front and the base of the skull in back. Head circumference is a particularly important measurement in infants up to about age six months. The head continues to grow after that, of course, but the chances of abnormality in head growth developing beyond that age are relatively small.

From age three on, you should measure the child's height and weight at least once every six months; it is no longer necessary to measure head circumference.

The National Center for Health Statistics has constructed growth charts for infants and children in the United States from infancy through age eighteen. These are based on the normal distribution curves mentioned earlier, though they are not themselves bell curves. Following are fourteen separate charts, each dealing with one aspect of growth—weight, length (stature), or head circumference. Stature is the same as length, the only difference being that stature refers to a child's height measured standing up, while length is the same measurement taken on an infant lying down. Each measurement is plotted in relation to age except for the last two charts, which compare weight with stature. There are separate charts for boys and girls.

How to Read a Growth Chart.   Refer to chart #1: Girl's Length by Age: Birth–36 Months. The baby's age in months is shown across the bottom, while the length is shown up the sides—length in centimeters on the right side and in inches on the left. (Each chart gives measurements in both metric and common English equivalents.) By following a growth line across the chart, you can trace the growth in length of a typical baby through the first three years. At age twelve months, for example, a typical baby girl might measure anywhere from 27.6 to 31 inches in length. This range of lengths is the normal variability which we talked about earlier.

There are seven different growth lines, or curves, on each chart representing the 5th, 10th, 25th, 50th, 75th, 90th, and 95th percentiles. Your child's growth should parallel one of these lines. The greatest number of children will grow along the 50th percentile line. A smaller number of children will grow along the 25th and 75th percentiles, and fewer still will grow along the 10th and 90th percentiles.

Chart 1. Girls' Length by Age: Birth—36 Months

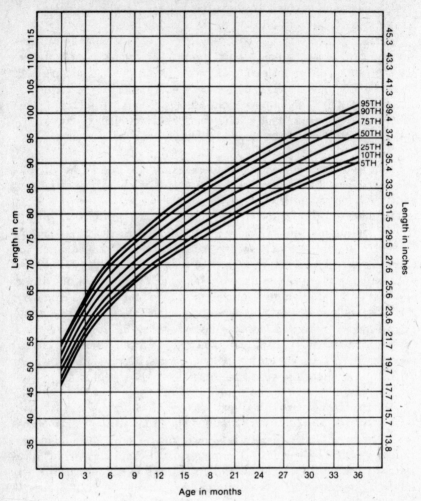

Chart 2. Boys' Length by Age: Birth–36 Months

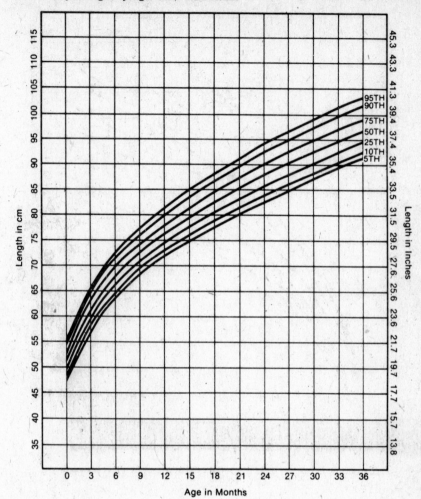

Chart 3. Girls' Weight by Age: Birth−36 Months

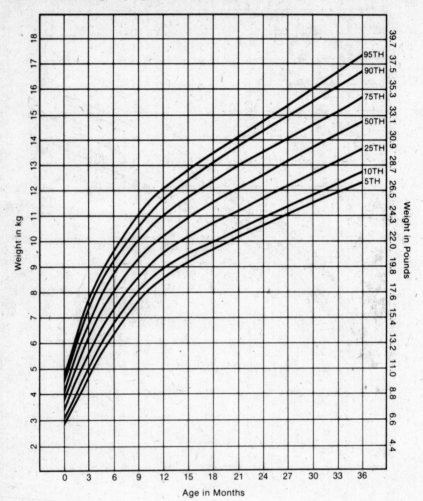

Chart 4. Boys' Weight by Age: Birth−36 Months

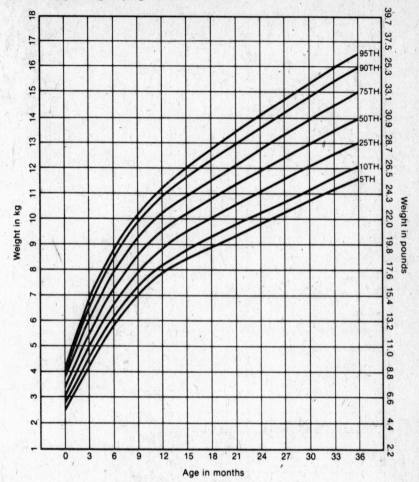

Chart 5. Girl's Head Circumference by Age: Birth–36 Months

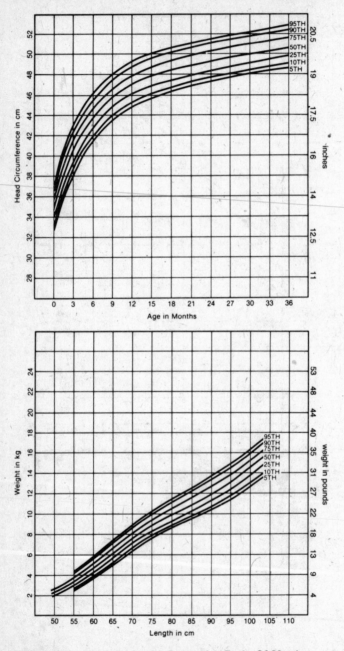

Chart 6. Girls' Weight by Length Percentiles: Birth–36 Months

Chart 7. Boys' Head Circumference by Age: Birth–36 Months

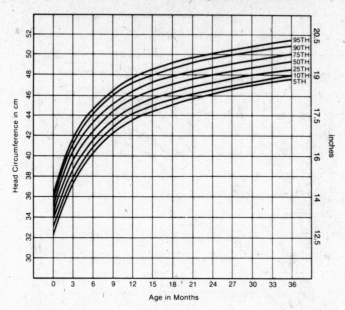

Chart 8. Boys' Weight by Length Percentiles: Birth–36 Months

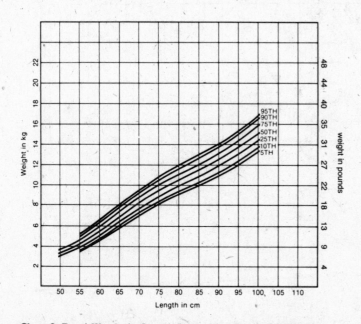

Chart 9. Girls' Stature by Age: 2 to 18 years.

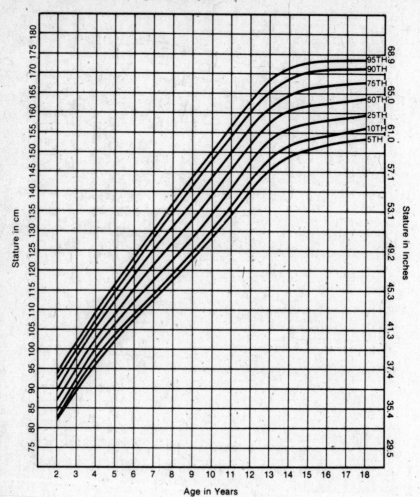

Chart 10. Boys' Stature by Age: 2 to 18 Years

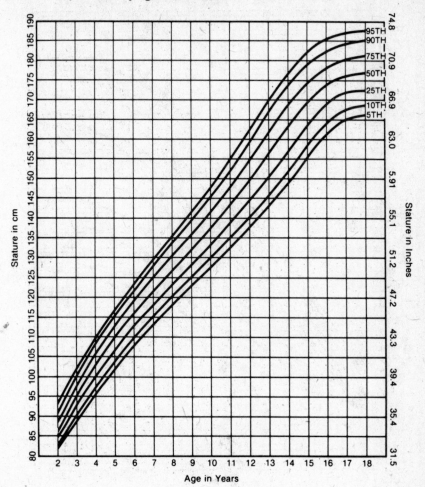

Chart 11. Girls' Weight by Age: 2 to 18 Years

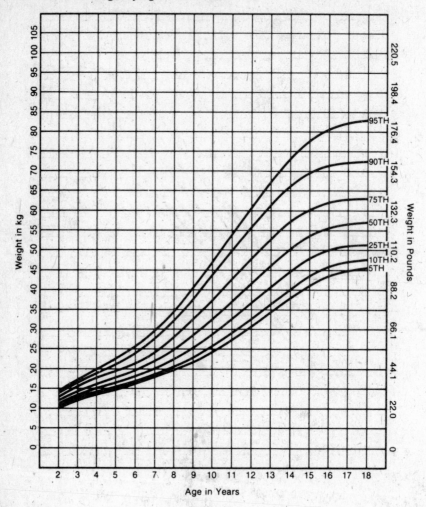

Chart 12. Boys' Weight by Age: 2 to 18 Years

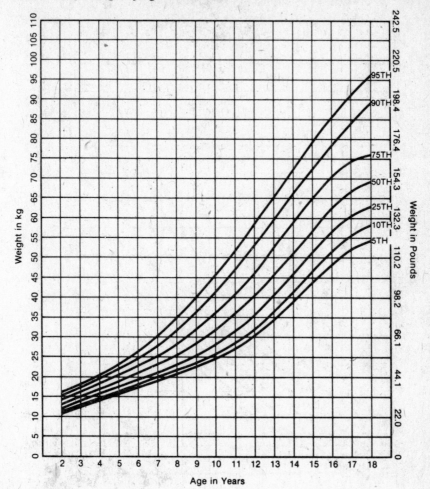

Chart 13. Weight by Stature for Prepubertal Girls

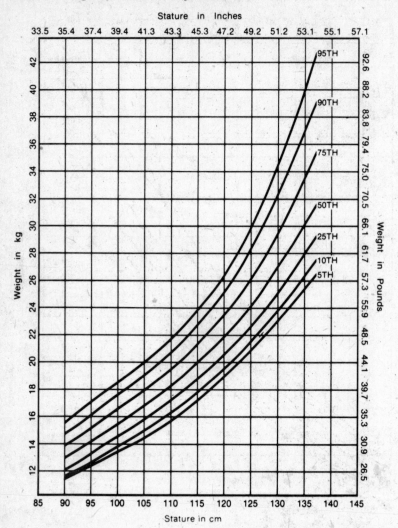

Chart 14. Weight by Stature for Prepubertal Boys

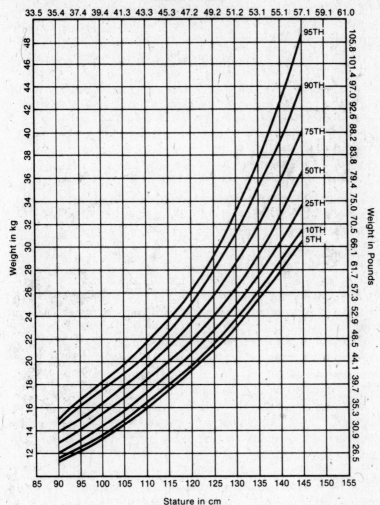

Stature in Inches

Children whose growth parallels the 5th percentile are unusually small in comparison with other children their age, and those who grow along the 95th percentile are unusually large for their age. Growth rates below the 5th or above the 95th percentiles are usually considered abnormal.

These charts were developed for use as a reference guide to assist doctors in detecting nutritional and growth disturbances in children. You can use them to plot your own child's growth and monitor his or her progress in comparison with the rest of the United States child population of the same age and sex.

Plotting Growth Statistics

The primary objective in monitoring a child's growth is to determine which of the standard growth curves your child is following. To do this, you must measure your child regularly and plot these growth statistics on the appropriate chart. Infants should be measured monthly using the procedure described earlier, and children over the age of three should be measured at least once every six months.

1. Record each measurement as you take it, making sure to label it correctly—for example, weight, length, or head circumference—and note the unit of measurement used—metric or common English.

2. Transfer each measurement to the appropriate chart. Find the child's age along the bottom of the chart and go up from there to the line corresponding to the measurement you have recorded. Make a mark here with a colored pen. If you are monitoring the growth of more than one child, use a different color for each child.

3. As the child grows and more measurements are plotted on the charts, connect the dots with a line of the same color. This is your child's growth line, and it should parallel one of the growth lines indicated on the chart.

Children will tend to follow the same percentile line for the bulk of their growing period. A small child following the 10th percentile line at age four will most likely still be following the 10th percentile line at age twelve. Similarly, a larger child following the 75th percentile line at age four will also be at that line at age twelve. This is true for both height and weight. If you find that your child is growing at a rate below the 5th or above the 95th percentiles, you should bring this fact to the attention of your doctor. You should also be concerned if a child growing along the 50th percentile line, for instance, suddenly stops growing as fast as the line indicates should be expected. During a serious illness, most children will tend to fall off their growth curve lines. If, after several repeated measurements, you are certain that your child is not following one of the standard growth curves, you should bring this fact to the attention of your doctor promptly.

SKELETAL ABNORMALITIES

A number of common skeletal deformities are not apparent at birth. Abnormalities involving the feet, legs, and hips often do not show up until the child starts walking, and spinal deformities in adolescents may be dismissed as poor posture and go untreated until the defect becomes painfully obvious. Many such problems can be readily corrected if the condition is treated early enough, and some may correct themselves. All too often, however, minor skeletal abnormalities such as pigeon toes or pronated ankles are not recognized until they interfere with normal growth and development. Here are some tests and observations you can use to detect such conditions in your child and bring them to the attention of your doctor before they cause trouble.

Metatarsus Varus.   The metatarsal bones in your feet connect the heel bones with the toe bones, and *varus* is a Latin word meaning

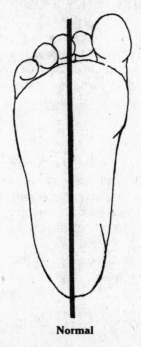
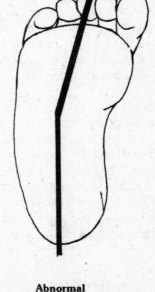

Normal   Abnormal

"bent inward." Metatarsus varus, then (also called metatarsus adductus), is an abnormal, inward curvature of the foot. The condition is usually apparent at birth, and can affect one or both feet.

Recognizing Metatarsus Varus

This condition is easy to recognize if you examine the soles of the baby's feet. Normally, a baby's feet should be straight from heel to toe so that if you draw a straight line up from the center of the heel, it will pass through the third toe, dividing the baby's foot in half. In metatarsus varus, however, the foot curves inward like a large comma, so that a line starting from the center of the heel would go through the two smallest toes at the outside of the foot. In this case, you would have to draw a *curved* line to connect the center of the heel and the third toe.

The simplest cases of metatarsus varus will correct themselves. If, however, the condition persists beyond the third or fourth month, you should bring this to the attention of your pediatrician. At this age, the condition can usually be corrected in a matter of weeks and it is important to straighten any curvature before the child starts walking.

Tibial Torsion.   The tibia is the main bone of the lower leg, and torsion simply means twisting. Thus, tibial torsion is a twisting of the lower leg.

A baby's legs are normally bowed at birth and will remain bowed until he or she begins to walk. Tibial torsion adds an inward twist to the normal bowing effect that causes the inner sole of the foot, where the arch will be, to turn sharply inward and upward toward the body. While the condition can occur in both legs, the left leg is more frequently affected than the right.

Checking for Tibial Torsion

Observe the position of the baby's legs when the infant is lying on its back. The legs will naturally assume a froglike position with the heels together and toes pointing slightly outward. Normally, if you bend the baby's knees and bring them together, the feet will point straight upwards. If tibial torsion is present, however, the foot of the affected leg will point inward when the knees are brought together.

Similarly, when the baby lies face down on a table, tibial torsion in one leg will cause both feet to point in the same direction, instead of pointing outward in opposite directions.

As in metatarsus varus, tibial torsion is apt to correct itself. Keep an

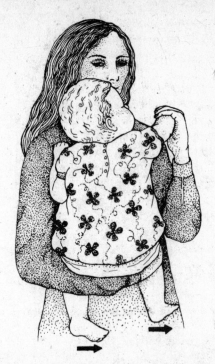

Tibial torsion causes both feet to point in the same direction.

eye on the condition, though, and if it does not show marked improvement by the age of five or six months, consult your pediatrician.

Femoral Torsion.   The femur is the upper leg bone and, like the tibia, it too can be twisted inward at birth. Femoral torsion almost always affects both legs, causing them to turn inward, limiting the normal range of motion.

Detecting Femoral Torsion
Have the child lie on his or her back with the legs fully extended and the feet pointing up. Normally, you should be able to rotate each foot about 15 degrees inward and about 60 degrees outward. In a child with femoral torsion, however, you will barely be able to turn the feet outward at all. Inward rotation, on the other hand, extends a full 90 degrees so that the inside of the foot, from heel to big toe, can be layed down flat.

This condition, too, usually straightens itself out eventually, which is fortunate because, unlike curvature of the tibia or the metatarsals, femoral torsion can only be corrected with massive surgery.

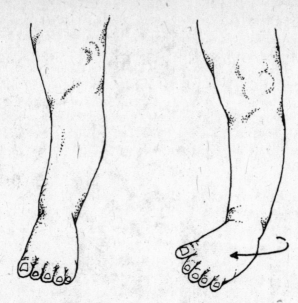

Tibial torsion causes the leg to turn sharply inward.

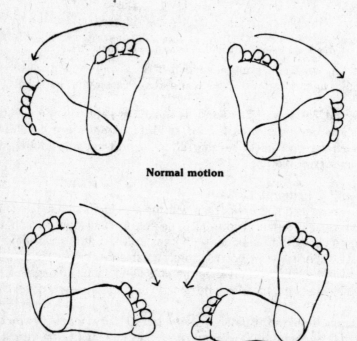

Normal motion

Femoral torsion

Pronated Ankles.   Pronation means to bend or turn face downward, and this is what pronated ankles do. In this condition, both ankles turn inward toward the ground. The problem becomes readily apparent after the child starts walking, at which time parents notice that he or she seems to have no arch. Flat feet in young children is generally not a cause for concern; usually, the arch is merely obscured by a normal pad of fat at the base of the arch which provides support until the bones harden and the muscles develop. Pronated ankles, on the other hand, are definitely abnormal and should be seen by a pediatrician.

Recognizing Pronated Ankles

Observe the child's legs from behind while he or she is standing up. Draw an imaginary line starting at the center of the heel and going straight up the leg. Normally, this line should bisect the middle of the heel, the heel cord, the center of the ankles, and the center of the knee. If the child has pronated ankles, however, your imaginary line from heel to knee will pass *outside* the ankle joint; the line would have to swerve inward at the ankle to bisect heel, ankle and knee.

If you think your child may have pronated ankles, you can confirm your suspicions by examining the pattern of wear of your child's shoes.

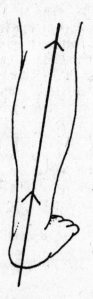

Normal

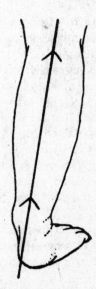

Pronated ankle

A child with pronated ankles will wear out a pair of shoes along the inside edge of the soles and heels. Similarly, the upper part of the shoes will be broken down along the inner side because of the excessive pressure exerted by the pronated ankles. This condition is generally corrected with special shoes, arch supports, and other devices prescribed by your pediatrician.

Congenital Dislocation of the Hip.　The hip joint is essentially a ball-and-socket arrangement in which the head of the femur, the upper leg bone, fits into the socket of the pelvis, or hip bone. In some infants this socket does not develop properly and is too shallow to hold the ball of the femur in place. Although the hip is equipped with the usual supply of ligaments binding the joint together, these tough, fibrous bands cannot compensate for the shallowness of the socket. Thus, when pressure is exerted at the joint, the ball of the femur tends to slip upward out of the socket, resulting in partial or complete dislocation of the hip.

Unless this deformity is detected in the routine examination of the infant in the first months of life, the condition may go unnoticed by parents until the child starts walking with a waddling gait. By this time, unfortunately, treatment is both difficult and unsatisfactory. The condition affects girls about five times as often as boys, and involves the left hip more frequently than the right.

Testing for Congenital Dislocation of the Hip

To check for this abnormality in an infant, lay the baby on its back and bring both knees up to the belly and then out to the sides, creating a 90-degree angle with the legs. If either hip joint is improperly developed, you will feel resistance and may feel or hear a snap, but don't push too hard. The affected side will have increased resistance.

A second test is to turn the infant over on its stomach and observe the backs of the thighs. A dislocated hip shortens that leg because the femur is resting above its normal position in the hip socket. This creates an extra fold of skin on the back of the thigh of the affected leg. If one hip is dislocated, you should be able to detect this extra fold of skin by carefully comparing the backs of both thighs.

Congenital dislocation of the hip is not painful to the infant, but it is nonetheless imperative that you bring such a condition to the attention of your doctor promptly as it will cause considerable trouble later in life.

Spinal Abnormalities.   The twenty-six vertebrae stacked one on top of another to make up our spinal column are dependent upon an intricate support structure made up of muscles, tendons, ligaments, and cartilage to maintain proper aligment (see "Understanding Your Back" in the chapter on bones, muscles, and joints). If any one of these elements fails to fulfill its support function, the spinal column will eventually suffer. In adults, the cartilaginous discs separating the vertebrae are common sources of trouble. In children, however, spinal abnormalities are generally seated in one of the basic muscle groups supporting the back.

These muscle groups act as guy wires, with each exerting the precise amount of pull necessary to hold the spinal column erect. Occasionally, one of these muscle groups may fail to develop properly. This can be due to a disease such as polio, a hereditary defect, or poor posture over a period of years, although more often than not the cause is unknown. Whatever the reason, when one muscle group weakens, another, stronger muscle group may pull the body out of line. This is what happens in scoliosis, which is a lateral (side-to-side) curvature of the spine. This condition is most likely to develop in children between the ages of ten and fifteen, with the incidence being much higher in girls and more common around age twelve or thirteen. No one knows exactly why it happens. As explained in the chapter "Bones, Muscles, and Joints," scoliosis can be corrected if caught in time. The condition "sets," however, at about age seventeen and treatment after that is likely to be more drastic and the final results less satisfactory. For this reason, we are including the test for scoliosis both here and in the chapter on "Bones, Muscles, and Joints." It is critically important that young people be examined regularly throughout their adolescent years for indications of scoliosis.

Detecting Scoliosis

There are several checks you can make that may help you detect scoliosis.

The first test involves a critical inspection of the subject's spinal column. Have the subject stand up straight with his or her back bared to just below the waist. The little knobby protrusions running down the center of the back are the spinous processes of the individual vertebrae. They should line up in a perfectly vertical column that does not deviate the least bit from side to side. Observe this column closely for signs of lateral curvature.

If you have any trouble locating the spinous processes, try this: Ask

the subject to bend forward slightly from the waist; this will make the
bony knobs more prominent. Then, using a black felt-tip pen, make a
little dot on the skin directly over each spinous process (there are 24).
When this is completed, have the subject again stand straight. The little
dots should form an absolutely straight line up the back.

A dropped shoulder is another indication of scoliosis. Observe the
subject standing up with his or her back to you, again bared to just
below the waist. Check to see that one shoulder does not drop lower
than the other. They should be equal.

A variation of this test is to have the subject stand with his or her feet
slightly apart and bend forward slowly at the waist, letting the arms hang
down in front and keeping the knees straight. As the upper body drops
downward, watch closely from behind to see if one side of the torso is
higher than the other at any time. Normally, both sides should remain
equal.

Lastly, you may be able to detect scoliosis in its very early stages by
recognizing an uneven development of the back muscles. Have the
subject lie on the floor, stomach down, with hands behind the neck.
Hold the subject's legs down and ask him or her to raise the upper body
off the floor so that the chest just clears the floor, and hold this position
for a moment or two. (*Caution:* Do not ask anyone who has been
experiencing back trouble to arch their back in this way.) This position
will exaggerate the muscles that run longitudinally along either side of
the spine. Lay your hand, palm down, over the muscles, first on one
side of the spine and then the other. The muscles should be equally
developed on both sides of the spine. Uneven development of the
spine's extensor muscles may indicate incipient scoliosis.

Rounded Back.   A rounded back is another spinal abnormality
occasionally seen in children. If not corrected with the appropriate
exercises, this condition can lead to headaches and stiffness and pain
through the shoulders and neck. You can check for a rounded back in
your child by critically observing his or her posture.

Observing Posture for Signs of Round-back

Try to observe your child's posture when he or she is not aware of it, as
minor defects can be disguised momentarily only to return when you
have finished your inspection.

Look first at the shoulders. Ideally, they should be straight and thrust
back, with the upper back flat and wide. The child with a rounded back,
on the other hand, looks hunched over as if he or she is drawing the
shoulders together in front. This abnormal curvature at the shoulders

throws the rest of the spine out of line as well. The round back extends up to the neck where it causes the head to bow forward a bit. Since this carriage effectively restricts the child's view in front, he or she compensates by stretching the neck forward and jutting the chin out. The resulting effect is that of a turtle emerging from its shell.

At the other end of the spine, the round back accentuates the natural inward curve (the lumbar lordosis) at the small of the back just above the buttocks. This exaggerated curve thrusts the abdomen out in front and the buttocks in back.

A rounded back all too often goes undiagnosed and uncorrected in young people for a variety of reasons. Parents may mistakenly assume that the youngster is slouching out of sheer perversity, or because it's the style among their friends. They may erroneously believe that the child will eventually grow out of it. Then, too, the condition develops so gradually that parents may not even notice the defect. A certain amount of objectivity is useful here. Sometimes it takes an outsider, such as a friend or relative who has not seen the child recently, to detect gradual changes in a young person's posture.

If you find yourself continually admonishing a child to stand up straight and stop slouching, consider the possibility that he or she may be unable to maintain correct posture because of a rounded back or other form of spinal curvature. If you suspect such a condition exists, you should bring this to the attention of your doctor without delay.

GROWTH OF TEETH

The Primary Teeth.   A common misconception about the primary teeth is that, because they are not permanent, they are not important. This attitude is extremely unfair to your baby. While the first set of teeth may be ultimately destined for the tooth fairy, they are nonetheless instrumental in paving the way for healthy permanent teeth. Healthy baby teeth guide the permanent teeth into their proper positions. Premature loss of the primary teeth due to decay or injury leaves unnatural gaps in the mouth. If other teeth are allowed to drift into these gaps, the permanent teeth will probably come in crooked. In the long run, the care you spend on your child's first teeth will be a worthwhile investment toward the permanent set.

In contrast to an adult set of thirty-two, a baby will eventually have just twenty teeth—ten in the upper jaw and ten in the lower. Starting in front, the primary teeth (also called milk teeth or deciduous teeth) include two central incisors flanked on either side by a lateral incisor, a canine and, finally, two molars at either end. This is the same in both jaws.

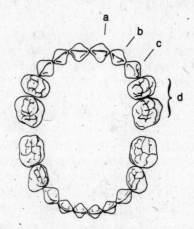

The Primary Teeth

(a) Central incisor, (b) lateral incisor, (c) canine, (d) molars.

The following chart shows the normal sequence of eruption and the average ages at which the primary teeth appear in most babies. The incisors are the first to erupt, followed by the first molars, the canines, and the second molars, with the teeth in the lower jaw generally appearing about six to eight weeks before their counterparts in the upper jaw. This timetable may vary in some children by as much as six months to a year and still be considered normal. Any greater deviation from this schedule should, however, be brought to the attention of the child's dentist.

ERUPTION AND LOSS OF PRIMARY TEETH

	Average Age of Eruption		
Type of Tooth	Lower	Upper	Average Age of Loss
Central incisors	6 months	7½ months	7th year
Lateral incisors	7 months	9 months	8th year
First molars	12 months	14 months	10th year
Canines (cuspids)	16 months	18 months	10th year
Second molars	20 months	24 months	11–12th year

Examining the Primary Teeth.   Starting at age two and a half, by which time all the primary teeth should be in, you should examine your child's teeth regularly every three months. The primary teeth should be examined in much the same way as the adult teeth, using the penlight and dental-mirror procedure described in the "Ears, Nose, Mouth, Throat, and Neck" chapter.

Many of the same problems that afflict adult teeth strike the baby teeth as well. Of these, dental decay is the most prevalent disease affecting the primary teeth. Newly erupted teeth are especially susceptible to decay. By the age of three, your child's teeth may already have cavities that require filling. You should also be alert to blows to the mouth such as might occur in a fall. As frequently happens in older children and adults, a well-directed blow to a tooth can kill the nerve and, consequently, the tooth itself. You should check for both of these conditions as instructed in the following tests in the "Ears, Nose, Mouth, Throat and Neck" chapter: "Checking for Cavities," "Testing for Plaque," and "Diagnosing Nerve Damage in a Tooth."

The First Permanent Molars.   Before your child loses the first baby tooth, the first permanent teeth will probably have erupted. This first permanent molar, also called the six-year molar because it usually appears around age six, erupts just behind the second baby molars. There is one on either side of each jaw for a total of four.

These molars have a special significance because they guide the placement of subsequent teeth. If they come in crooked, there's a good chance that others will, too. To avoid this, you should monitor this tooth's eruption as described below.

Monitoring the First Permanent Molars
The first permanent molars usually erupt between five and six and a half years of age. Well before they appear, however, you should inspect the baby molars.

1. Checking the primary molars: Just as the first permanent molars guide the placement of subsequent teeth, so do the primary molars guide in these six-year molars. By age five at the latest, check to see that all eight primary molars (two at either end of the jaw, top and bottom) are in view and are positioned properly. If any primary molars appear crooked, you should consult your dentist.
2. Watching for the first permanent molars: Beginning around age five, you should periodically check the gum tissue behind the baby molars for signs of the first permanent molars. Occasionally, one of

these teeth erupts through the gum, leaving a flap of tissue beneath which food particles can collect. When this happens, the gums can become sore and infected. In such cases, the dentist may choose to cut away the offending flap of tissue.

When these molars do erupt, check their placement and positioning. If the first permanent molars come in straight, chances are the rest of the permanent teeth will, too. If, however, any of these six-year molars appear crooked to you, you should bring this to the attention of your dentist.

Once the six-year molars are in, the rest of the permanent teeth should emerge pretty uneventfully. Here, in order of their eruption, is a chart telling when you can expect the rest. The baby molars, by the way, are replaced not by adult molars but by the bicuspids (also called

(a) Central incisor, (b) lateral incisor, (c) canine, (d) first bicuspid, (e) second bicuspid, (f) first molar, (g) second molar, (h) third molar.

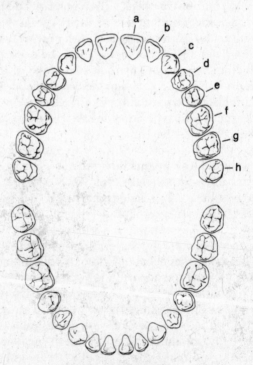

The Permanent Teeth

the premolars). As with the primary teeth, the ages at eruption may vary by several months either way.

ERUPTION OF PERMANENT TEETH

Type of Tooth	Average Age of Eruption	
	Lower	Upper
First molars	6th–7th year	6th–7th year
Central incisors	6th–7th year	7th–8th year
Lateral incisors	7th–8th year	8th–9th year
Canines (cuspids)	9th–10th year	11th–12th year
First bicuspids (premolars)	10th–12th year	10th–11th year
Second bicuspids (premolars)	11th–12th year	10th–12th year
Second molars	11th–13th year	12th–13th year
Third molars (wisdom)	17th–21st year	17th–21st year

DEVELOPMENTAL MILESTONES

A newborn baby is a bundle of reflexes. Touch an infant's cheek with your finger and the rooting reflex will prompt the baby to swivel its head around and take your finger in its mouth; then the sucking reflex goes into action. Pull an infant to a sitting position and its eyes will open like a china doll's (doll's eye reflex) and the baby will instinctively try to hold its head in an upright position (righting reflex). Some reflexes are precursors of later skills such as crawling and walking. If you place an infant on its belly, it will make rudimentary crawling movements; hold it in a standing position and the baby will demonstrate the stepping reflex.

There are a great many such reflexes governing everything from eye movements to bowel movements. In fact, much of an infant's behavior in the first two months is instinctual. As a baby adds pounds and inches, however, these reflex actions are replaced by voluntary movements that the baby can control at will—things like eye coordination, head control, balance, and later, walking and talking.

All of this progress unfolds in an orderly fashion, with each new feat building on previous achievements. People who study this developmental process have been able to chart the average ages at which most babies exhibit a particular mannerism or reach a specified goal. These "developmental milestones," as they are called, can be anything from a social smile to the first word. Since they occur at roughly the same age in most children, you can use this information to assess your own child's development.

However, just as there are wide variations in the normal height and weight of children at any given age, so too do developmental skills progress at different rates. Generally, the more complicated the task, the greater the normal range of variability. For instance, the first smile generally appears within a two-month span, whereas sitting up has a four-month variability range and walking can vary by as much as seven months from one child to another. Similarly, verbal ability may sprout in normal children at any time from twelve months to two years.

Clearly, then, the child who does not conform to an "average" pattern is not necessarily abnormal. Furthermore, rapid development in the first years of life does not guarantee superior intelligence later on. Children tend to develop in spurts, and the slow child this year is apt to outstrip his precocious friend next year. The purpose of the following outline is to present the sequence in which various skills are acquired and suggest some general guidelines as to when you might expect them. If your child consistently lags in reaching these developmental milestones, you should discuss this with a pediatrician.

Developmental Milestones, Birth Through Age Five

First four weeks. When lying on its back, baby generally pulls up the knees a bit, bends its arms, and clenches its fists. If baby is lifted to a sitting position, the head will tend to sag. Some but not all babies may fix their eyes on their mother's face or on a light which is directly in their line of vision. If held upright, he or she will tend to make stepping motions when the feet are placed against the floor or the crib mattress. The baby will also exhibit a startle response to a hand vigorously slapped against the mattress next to him (Moro reflex). The Moro reflex is a widely trusted test used by pediatricians. A poor Moro is an early sign of possible neurologic damage.

Two months. By eight weeks most babies can follow a moving object with the eyes, react to parents' voices, and smile in response to social contact.

Three months. Some head control should be evident at this point. When placed on the stomach, the baby should begin to lift its head off the mattress. If held in the air in a horizontal position with the stomach down, the baby will lift its head rather than allow it to droop. Some degree of head control is also demonstrated when the baby is pulled to a sitting position. Head control at this age is not yet very good, however. By twelve weeks most babies will listen to music and make rudimentary verbal sounds.

Four months. By this time the baby should have developed good head control when pulled to a sitting position. At sixteen weeks most babies will laugh out loud, reach out for an object with the hands (and probably miss), and display excitement at the sight of food at meal-times.

Seven months. Most babies are able to roll over by themselves from front to back and back to front. They are usually able to sit alone for very brief periods by leaning forward on the hands with the back rounded. Seven-month-old babies will usually reach out for objects offered to them, transfer an object from one hand to the other, and invariably bang it up and down on the tabletop. Language development continues, with most babies being able to make vowel sounds and sounds of several syllables. Babies this age can also drink from a mug with help, and will smile at their reflection in a mirror.

Eight to ten months. Around this time the average baby can sit alone, back straight, without toppling over. Most are able to crawl on hands and knees, or propel themselves along with sort of a hitching motion. Babies this age will uncover toys hidden beneath a cloth, and will use a thumb-and-forefinger (pincer) grasp instead of the more primitive palm grasp to pick up a small object. Social responsiveness is also heightened—by ten months most babies respond to the sound of their name, play simple games like peek-a-boo and pat-a-cake, and will reach out to be picked up. Vocabulary at this point typically consists of repetitive sounds such as ma-ma, da-da, and bye-bye.

Starting at age one year, child development is generally divided into four areas: motor (locomotion), adaptive (finer learned skills), language, and social.

Twelve months. Motor: Stands alone, walks with help. Adaptive: Picks up a bead using the thumb and forefinger and releases this object to another person upon request or gesture. Language: Speaks one or two words other than ma-ma or da-da. These are not necessarily standard or understandable words in the usual sense, but are more likely the child's own private language. Children often develop a small vocabulary of totally private words for common things such as water. Social: Plays simple ball games such as rolling and returning; makes some attempt to cooperate when being dressed.

Fifteen months. Motor: Walks alone, though occasionally a normal child will not walk until sixteen or seventeen months. Failure to walk until after eighteen months of age may be a sign of trouble. Adaptive: Able to make a tower by stacking one block on top of another; able to draw some kind of a line with a crayon; and can put a small toy or bit of candy like an M&M into a container. Language: Private vocabulary continues, but standard names for familiar objects such as cup and ball may be included in the vocabulary. Children at this age will usually begin to follow simple commands. Social: Begins to make needs known by pointing or by tugging at someone.

Eighteen months. Motor: Able to sit in a small chair, may be able to run, though quite stiffly, and walk upstairs with one hand held. Adaptive: Scribbles with a crayon, makes a three-block tower, and dumps small objects from a container. Language: Able to name a few objects from pictures and has a small vocabulary of five to ten understandable words.

Two years. Motor: Runs well and is able to walk both up and down stairs one step at a time. Also opens doors, climbs furniture, and generally has full mobility. Adaptive: Able to stack blocks to make a tower six blocks high; begins imitative writing behavior by scribbling in circles and making vertical and horizontal strokes. Language: May make simple, three-word sentences. Social: Handles spoon well, helps to undress, and listens to stories with pictures.

Two and one-half years. Motor: Runs, jumps, and goes up and down stairs one at a time. Adaptive: Able to stack a tower eight blocks high, though this task may take some encouragement and patience. Language: Uses the personal pronoun "I" correctly and knows full name. Social: Begins to be helpful in housekeeping tasks.

Three years. Motor: Uses alternating feet on stairs; rides tricycle. Adaptive: Builds a nine-block tower and constructs a three-block, bridge-type structure. Language: Knows age and sex, counts three objects correctly, and can repeat three numbers. Social: Plays simple games but does not yet actually play with a child of the same age. There is parallel play but very little game interaction. Helps with buttons and putting on shoes.

Four years. Motor: Hops on one foot, uses scissors to cut out pictures, climbs well, throws ball accurately. Adaptive: Able to complete a two-piece puzzle in less than four seconds and a three-piece puzzle in forty-five seconds or less. Can copy simple figures such as a cross and a square using a pencil or crayon, and draws a recognizable human figure. Language: Tells simple stories. Social: Plays with several other children in a socially interactive fashion.

Five years. Motor: Skips, hops, and jumps easily; able to catch a small ball. Adaptive: Copies simple geometric figures accurately, including square, triangle, and cross. Language: Names four colors, counts up to ten pennies accurately. Social: Dresses and undresses self, engages in household role-playing.

By age six, children are generally enrolled in school. Public school

systems in most states today are required to provide appropriate educational attention for special-needs children. As part of this program, a wide variety of developmental testing is usually carried out to identify these students. If you are concerned about your child's development at this point, you can ask that such tests be administered and the results made available to you. If your child is diagnosed as having a learning disability in some area, you should see that his or her special needs are met by the school.

DETECTING ILLNESS IN INFANTS AND CHILDREN

It takes a special talent sometimes to recognize an ill child, which is why a good pediatrician combines the training of a doctor with the instincts of a parent and the intuition of a mind reader. Instinct and intuition may seem like rather unscientific elements to base a diagnosis on, but then children are notoriously imprecise in describing where it hurts. They may say they have a headache when they actually have an earache, a toothache or even a stomachache. Pediatricians develop a sort of sixth sense about illness in children, and it generally serves them well. A pediatrician may say that a child looks ill even before the exact nature of the illness is determined. The simple fact that the child *seems* unwell will often prompt a doctor to carry out more vigorous diagnostic studies.

You may not have the professional training of a pediatrician, but you are probably the most astute observer of your child's well-being simply because you know him or her so intimately. Every child has certain mannerisms—moods, personal preferences, ways of moving, ways of talking—that a parent recognizes as normal. Small changes in a child's characteristic behavior are often valuable signs that something is wrong. And, of course, there are more concrete tests and observations that are helpful.

Fever. One of the most useful signs of illness in children is fever. Fever is an elevation of the body temperature in response to infection, either bacterial or viral. Monitoring a child's fever can provide you and the doctor with valuable information about your child's condition.

If your child seems ill, a temperature check is always a good first step. Body temperature can be measured using three methods—oral, rectal, or axillary—as follows.

Taking the Temperature of an Infant or Small Child

1. *Rectal temperature.* Body temperature should be taken in the

rectum of babies and small children who are unable to reliably hold an oral thermometer in the mouth. The rectal thermometer has a more bulbous-shaped mercury sensor than the oral thermometer.

To take a rectal temperature, place a small amount of petroleum jelly on the mercury tip of the thermometer and gently insert it a short way into the child's rectum. If the bulb is ½ to 1 inch beyond the opening of the rectum, this is quite adequate. A rectal reading registers rather quickly. Once inserted in the rectum, the mercury begins rising almost immediately; when it stops moving, within a minute or so, remove the thermometer.

A good technique to use on infants or uncooperative toddlers is to lay the child, bottom up, on your lap or on a table. Placing the heel of your left hand (or, if you are left-handed, your right hand) on the child's buttocks, spread them apart with your fingers, taking care to keep the child's legs flat so the knees don't work their way under the body. Now gently insert the tip of the thermometer with your free hand, maintaining your hold on the child's buttocks while the thermometer is in place.

2. *Oral temperature.* By age five or six years, most children will be able to reliably hold an oral thermometer in the mouth. In taking the temperature at this site, you must be certain that the bulb end of the thermometer is actually kept under the tongue and that the child does not bite the instrument. Instruct the child to breathe through the nose while the thermometer is in place. Three minutes' time is generally sufficient to register an accurate oral reading.

3. *Axillary temperature.* The axillary temperature refers to the body temperature at the armpit. This is taken by placing the thermometer as high as possible up under the child's armpit. The arm is then held firmly to the side while the thermometer remains in place for three to four minutes.

Of the three methods, the rectal temperature is the most reliable reflection of the actual internal temperature of the body. The oral temperature is the second most reliable, and the axillary runs a poor third. The normal rectal temperature is approximately one degree higher than the normal oral temperature, and the axillary temperature is about one degree (F.) lower than the oral temperature. When recording temperature it is therefore important to record not only the reading on the thermometer but the method by which the measurement was made—that is, oral, rectal, or axillary. When reporting a child's body temperature to a physician, do not add or subtract a degree in an attempt to make the temperature comparable to an oral reading. This may only confuse the doctor. Simply report the numbers and the location.

Once you have taken your child's temperature, the next step is to interpret your findings. To begin with, don't be misled by the little arrow pointing at 98.6°F. This supposedly "normal" body temperature is simply a mathematical average which, like average weights, heights, and other such figures, represents many but not all individuals. Your child's normal body temperature may very well be a bit higher or a bit lower than 98.6°. In fact, it's a good idea to take your child's temperature several times when he or she is feeling well, and record this figure in your child's health history. This will provide you with a reference figure against which to interpret subsequent readings.

Keep in mind, too, that fevers in children tend to be more dramatic than fevers in adults. Children sometimes run amazingly high fevers with relatively minor illnesses. Whereas a temperature of 102°F. usually indicates substantial illness in an adult, the same is not necessarily true for children. Even short-lived viral infections such as the flu produce fevers as high as 104° in children.

Thus the mere fact that the child is running a temperature is not in itself cause for serious alarm. The presence of fever can, however, be a revealing indicator of the child's condition when used as follows:

Evaluating the Significance of a Fever

1. *Response to aspirin.* A relatively reliable method of testing the severity of a fever in children is their response to aspirin. If a child develops a fever of up to 104°, administer a dose of aspirin or one of the nonaspirin, fever-reducing medicines and take the temperature again in an hour or so. If the child has a relatively mild (usually viral) illness, the temperature is likely to fall approximately one to one and one-half degrees and the child will both feel and act much better. Often children with this kind of illness will lie quietly in bed and look quite ill before you administer the aspirin, only to be running around the house two hours later. Children with more serious infections, on the other hand, do not generally show this kind of dramatic good response to aspirin. While their temperatures may fall in response to the medication, the child will not feel or behave noticeably better.

2. *Tracking fever.* An elevated body temperature in a child is more significant if monitored over the course of the illness. As soon as you realize that the child is feverish, keep a running record of body temperature over the next several days. Take the temperature twice a day and label your readings according to the method and time of day

they were taken—morning, afternoon, evening. Temperatures taken in the afternoon tend to be higher than morning or evening readings. Be sure to use the same method each time.

If over the course of a few days your child's temperature begins to climb after remaining relatively stable, or returns after having once subsided, this is an indication that the infection may have spread to a secondary site—such as from the throat to the ears—and you should consult a doctor.

Children with fevers higher than 103°F., or persistent and prolonged fever at any level, should be seen by a doctor. Even if the fever is well below 103° but you think your child is seriously ill, or if he or she is trembling with fever, see your doctor. And any fever at all in an infant younger than four months should be brought to the attention of your pediatrician.

Pain.   Pain is often a very elusive thing to pin down. Think back to the last time you were in pain. You probably complained in such vague terms as, "Gee, I don't feel so hot today." If pressed, you might have elaborated by saying, "Well, my arm has been bothering me." And if you had stopped to analyze it, you might have concluded that the pain was centered more precisely in the shoulder, not the arm, and thus narrowed down the source of your trouble to the joint.

Young children, on the other hand, are incapable of this kind of analytical reasoning. For one thing, they may not know the right words to express their pain. If they hurt once before and it was called a sore throat, they may call anything a sore throat now because, to them, this is a general term covering all varieties of pain and discomfort. In their impatience to get relief, they become short-tempered and irrational. They may complain of a headache while clutching their stomach, and generally make misleading, confusing, and contradictory statements until all you know for sure is that something, somewhere, hurts.

While a child in pain cannot be expected to diagnose his condition for you, there are a number of steps you can take to help both you and the child zero in on where it hurts.

Finding Out Where It Hurts

1. *Inspect.* Before subjecting a crying child to any lengthy examination, make a cursory inspection of his or her body to see if there is an obvious physical reason for discomfort. A stone in the shoe, a sliver in a hand or foot, a black-and-blue mark, an insect bite, and so on

are all common hurts that might be troubling your toddler. Have the child walk a few steps and watch for a limp or other abnormality in gait that might point to the problem. Once you have ruled out such obvious possibilities, you will have to question the child for additional information.

2. *Question.* A child in pain is in no mood to chat. But since he or she is the only person who knows where it hurts, the child is the logical party to consult.

It is important to understand, however, that it is very easy to come to an erroneous conclusion on the basis of a small child's responses. Many children will say what they think their parents want to hear. Then, too, a persuasive parent may actually convince the child he has a stomachache when the pain is really in his ear. Children are very susceptible to suggestion, so you must take care to frame your questions in such a way that an answer is not implied by the question.

For instance, instead of asking "Is your tummy upset?" "Do you have a sore throat?" or "Does your head hurt?" phrase your questions so that the child has to supply his own response, not just echo yours. Questions like "How does your tummy feel?" and "Point to where it hurts" are more likely to yield reliable information. If you suspect a sore throat is the problem, a question like "How does it feel when you swallow?" may elicit a revealing answer.

If the child is old enough, it might be helpful to review the day's activities for clues to the present discomfort. What have they had to eat? Where have they been? What games did they play? Did they fall down or get hit by anything in the course of their recent activities? Encourage the child to think back to the day before. Be alert for answers which may suggest food poisoning, a mild concussion, or just simple indigestion.

3. *Examine.* By this point you should have some idea of where the trouble lies. If so, a brief examination may help you determine the nature of the problem.

Abdominal pain should be localized—that is, pinpointed—with a series of questions. To do this, ask the child to lie on his or her back and place your hand over various areas of the abdomen, asking the child where it hurts most. A detailed discussion of the abdomen and the various organs located in each of the four quadrants is presented in the chapter "Tracing and Testing the Digestive Process."

If the child complains of pain in an extremity, it is important to examine the entire extremity before concluding that any one part is causing the problem. For example, children with a disorder of the hip are often brought to the physician with a complaint that something is wrong with the child's knee and he or she is limping. A careful examination, however, may reveal a limited range of motion of the hip and considerable pain on moving the hip into certain positions, whereas the knee is freely mobile and pain-free.

Once you have narrowed down the probable source of a child's pain, you will be in a much better position to evaluate its significance and, if necessary, more accurately report the child's condition to the doctor.

The evaluation of nausea, vomiting, abdominal pain, and bowel problems is particularly difficult in school-age children. Children with minor adjustment problems or emotional disorders will often express them as stomach or abdominal ailments. In such children a complaint that "I have a stomachache" may mean that there is a pain somewhere in the abdomen, or it may mean that the child does not want to go to school that day. Dealing with this sort of situation requires patience, insight, and understanding. Children frequently develop school phobias and shrink from certain activities or situations for reasons even they themselves may not understand. There may be a bad situation with a teacher or friend or, more likely, an overwhelming fear of failure in the face of others the child admires. Unable to deal with the stressful situation, the child develops vague or even specific abdominal pain, nausea, vomiting, or urgency to have a bowel movement. Despite their intangible basis, these psychosomatic complaints can be very real for the child.

Since any of these symptoms may indicate true organic disease as well as the outward manifestation of an emotional problem, evaluating their significance is at the same time difficult and important. Several points may be helpful, here. First, if the disorder is psychosomatic in nature, the child is much less likely to look really sick than if the disease has an organic cause such as internal injury or infection. Organic disease severe enough to cause vomiting, diarrhea, or substantial abdominal pain usually affects the child's behavior in such a way that he or she appears unmistakably ill to a parent. This is not an absolutely hard and fast rule, but it is helpful. Secondly, the timing of the event is important. If the child regularly complains of such symptoms each morning just before going to school but not on Saturday or Sunday or during holiday periods, it is most likely that the problem is psychosomatic rather than organic. If the symptoms happen only at school and always at the same time of day, this should provide an even better clue as to what it is in the school situation that is disturbing the child. There is virtually no important, strictly organic disease which induces nausea, vomiting, abdominal pain, or diarrhea on school days and not on Saturday or Sunday.

While medication can be helpful in controlling some of the symptoms of these psychosomatic disorders, the only real cure comes when the reasons for the child's unhappiness are brought to the surface and dealt with.

If your child develops recurrent complaints of almost any sort, it is wise to keep a record noting the date, time of day and severity of the symptoms. A pattern of occurrences is likely to emerge and this can be very helpful to the physician in dealing with the problem.

IDENTIFYING PERCEPTION PROBLEMS IN SMALL CHILDREN

Vision.   By age four or five, most children's eyesight can be tested at home using an eye chart (the "E" chart) as described in the chapter "Testing Vision." A special version of this test designed for home use by parents of preschoolers is available at no charge from The National Society for the Prevention of Blindness, 79 Madison Avenue, New York, NY 10016.

Even before testing your child's visual acuity, however, you should test for two other conditions that may threaten his or her vision. One is strabismus, or "squint," and the other is amblyopia, better known as "lazy eye," and both can lead to serious vision impairment if not detected and treated at an early age.

Strabismus.   Strabismus is an abnormality involving the eye muscles that makes it difficult to coordinate eye movements. Each eye perceives a slightly different image, causing the child to "see double." Since double vision is very uncomfortable, the child learns to "tune out" one of the images. This in turn can lead to amblyopia (see below).

Strabismus is also known as turned eyes because of the characteristic effect produced when one eye turns in or out. Very early strabismus, in the first two to three months, may correct itself. By age six months, however, the eyes should be coordinating correctly. If you are uncertain whether your baby's eyes are properly coordinated, you should check for strabismus with this simple flashlight test.

Testing for Strabismus
Hold a flashlight about two feet in front of the baby's face and shine the

light briefly into the eyes. Observe the child's eyes closely to see where the light is reflected in the eyes. Normally, if the baby is staring directly into the light, its reflection should be located in the very center of each pupil. If the baby is looking away from the light, the reflection should strike at the same spot on the iris (colored part) of each eye.

If, however, the eyes do not focus properly because of strabismus, the reflection of the flashlight will strike the eyes at different spots—such as the pupil of one eye and some point on the colored part of the other.

If you suspect that your child may have strabismus, you should have his or her eyes checked by an ophthalmologist without delay. Age one is not too young to begin correcting strabismus, and after age three may be too late.

Amblyopia.   Amblyopia is a vision defect in which one eye sees better than the other. Sometimes the condition is due to a "turned eye"—strabismus—that causes double vision. But just as frequently there are no obvious defects that might alert parents to the problem. In any event, the stronger eye, because it sees better, is used more than the weaker eye. Eventually, vision in the "lazy" eye is lost as a result of disuse.

If detected by age three, most cases of amblyopia respond well to treatment. Success rates decline in older children, however. Unfortunately, most children's eyesight is first tested in the schools, by which time the effects of amblyopia may well be irreversible. For this reason, you should administer the following test to your toddler by age three, or as soon as the child is capable of taking the test.

Testing for Amblyopia

1. You will need a wide, black felt-tip marking pen and six unlined 3 × 5 index cards. In the center of each card, draw one of the following figures: ice cream cone, star, daisy, house, happy face, sad face. Make your drawings about one-half inch high and as simple as possible so that the child will have no difficulty recognizing each figure.

2. Show each of the six cards to the child and go over them with him or her, identifying each one at close range with both eyes.

3. Show the child how to cover one eye with a paper cup.

4. Stand ten feet away from the child. Ask the child to cover one eye and hold the cards up one at a time for him or her to identify. If the child cannot recognize the figures at this distance, move forward until he or

she can and note the greatest distance at which the child can identify the figures on the cards.

5. Now test the other eye following the same procedure.

6. Compare your results. A difference of three feet or more in the distance at which each eye can identify the figures on the cards may indicate a "lazy" eye.

Hearing.   A hearing loss has far-reaching effects on a child. Most obvious is the absence of speech. Babies learn to speak by imitating the sounds they hear spoken to them. Babies who do not hear do not begin talking. Less obvious is the effect of a hearing loss on the child's personality. Children who cannot hear are effectively isolated from the mainstream of activity, and the resulting loneliness is compounded by the frustration of being unable to communicate their needs and feelings.

Every parent should be alert to signs of a hearing problem in their baby. Particular attention should be paid to this aspect of a child's development when (1) there is a family history of hearing loss, (2) there is an Rh or other blood group incompatibility, (3) the mother had German measles (rubella), a high fever, or some viral infection during the first three months of pregnancy, or (4) there were complications during delivery.

Even before a baby should be talking, you may be able to detect a hearing disability by closely observing his or her behavior, as follows.

Detecting Hearing Loss in Infants

Certain aspects of a baby's development depend on the ability to hear. You can check your baby's hearing by observing his or her behavior at various stages of development for these characteristic responses to sounds.

Birth to 3 months.   Is startled by loud sounds; is soothed by mother's voice.

3 to 6 months.   Turns eyes and head to search for location of sound; listens to conversations; imitates his own noises—oohs, ba-ba's, and so on; enjoys rattles and other sound-making toys.

6 to 10 months.   Responds to his own name, hears a ringing telephone; understands common words such as "no," "hot," and "bye-bye."

10 to 15 months.   Obeys simple commands such as "come!"; points to familiar objects or persons when asked to do so; speaks first words.

15 to 18 months.   Follows simple spoken directions; has a vocabulary of several words.

If your baby consistently fails to meet these developmental milestones, you should have his or her hearing checked by an otologist without delay.

Learning Disabilities.   Just about every child experiences academic plateaus and setbacks of one kind or another during their school years. These may be due to anything from illness and injury to emotional problems and competing interests. Usually they are transitory and the child eventually catches up with the rest of the class once the underlying conflict has been worked out.

For one reason or another, however, some children find it extremely trying to master skills and concepts that others pick up with ease. When they enter school, they have difficulty adjusting to the structured environment of the typical classroom. And as time goes on, they fall further and further behind until their failure to learn takes its toll on their self-esteem. When this happens, they may doubt their own ability to learn and eventually give up trying.

Many such children are wrongly stigmatized by parents and teachers as retarded, unmanageable, or just plain troublesome when the problem is actually a learning disability stemming from brain-function processes that are not yet fully understood.

Children with learning disabilities often have average or above average intelligence, yet they encounter significant learning difficulties. Perception problems such as dyslexia, in which the child has trouble differentiating between letters and words that are mirror images of one another—such as *b* and *d, on* and *no, saw* and *was*—may interfere with reading progress. Poor coordination may show up in the child's handwriting and on the playground. Children with learning disabilities may have a normal range of hearing, yet confuse similar sounding words such as book and brook when they hear them spoken. Parents and teachers alike invariably describe such youngsters as impulsive, hyperactive, and easily distracted, with a memory like a sieve.

But don't jump to the conclusion that your child has a learning disability simply because he or she won't sit still and never listens to you. Alas, 'twas ever thus! You should, however, think in terms of a learning disability if your child consistently fails to keep up with his or her class, both academically and socially.

The following sets of questions were devised by The New York Institute for Child Development to alert parents to a possible learning disability in their child. If you answer yes to at least ten (20 percent) of the questions in the appropriate age group—preschool, grades 1–8, or high school—it may be that your child has a learning disability. If so, you should contact your child's school to arrange for further testing and remedial help geared to his or her individual needs.

Learning Disabilities Checklist*

Preschool Age: 4—5

1. Is your child afraid of heights? (i.e., won't climb on jungle jim; doesn't like to be picked up)
2. Is your child extremely daring?
3. Is your child easily distractible?
4. Is your child always up and down from the table during meals?
5. Is your child a discipline problem?
6. Does your child seem to "tune-out" at times?
7. Does your child find it necessary to touch everything he/she sees?
8. Does your child frequently walk into things or trip?
9. Is there inconsistency in your child's performance? (i.e., one day he/she performs a task well, the next day he/she can't)
10. Does your child have a short attention span?
11. Does your child get frequent headaches?
12. Does your child frustrate easily?
13. Does your child have difficulty keeping rhythm while dancing or clapping?
14. Is your child unusually sensitive to light, noise, touch, or certain clothing material?
15. Was your child a late walker?
16. Was your child a prolonged tiptoe walker?
17. Was your child's speech late or abnormal?
18. Does your child have frequent nightmares?
19. Is your child a bedwetter?
20. Does your child have uncontrollable rage reactions?
21. Does your child complain of seeing things bigger or smaller than they are?
22. Is your child always tired?
23. Is your child unable to keep up with the other children's activity levels?
24. Does your child have a poor appetite?
25. Does your child have a history of anemia of any type?
26. Is your child irritable before and/or shortly after meals?

*Reprinted with the permission of The New York Institute for Child Development.

27. Is your child easily fatigued?

28. Does your child exhibit excessive thirst?

29. Does your child crave sweets?

30. Has your child experienced excessive weight gain or loss?

31. Did your child have trouble learning to skip?

32. Does it seem that your child never pays attention to you?

33. Is your child unable to modulate his/her voice?

34. Does your child keep his/her head very close to the paper or tilt it back and forth when reading or writing?

35. Does your child have frequent stomachaches?

36. Does your child frequently go out of the lines when coloring?

37. Did your child have trouble learning how to tie and/or button and/or lace?

38. Does your child always seem to have a cold?

39. Was your child colicky?

40. Was your child an unusually cranky baby?

41. Was your child an unusually passive baby?

42. Does your child do everything to excess? (i.e., laugh, cry, talk, sleep, perspire)

43. Does your child have poor bowel or bladder control?

44. Does your child seem preoccupied with matches, fire, etc.?

45. Is your child a bully?

46. Is your child always picked on by his/her peers?

47. Is your child a loner?

48. Does your child's walking or running seem clumsy or disjointed?

49. Is your child ever purposely destructive?

50. Does your child have a history of allergies?

Grades 1–8

1. Does your child have difficulty understanding what he/she reads?

2. Does your child avoid sports or activities that involve catching and throwing a ball?

3. Is your child very afraid of heights? (i.e., won't climb on the jungle jim; doesn't like to be picked up)

4. Is your child extremely daring?

5. Does your child's running seem uncoordinated or sloppy?

6. Does your child get lost frequently?

7. Is your child easily distractible?

8. Does your child confuse right from left?

9. Does your child use one hand for some things and the other hand for other things?

10. Is your child always up and down from the table during meals?

11. Is your child a discipline problem?

12. Does your child go up or down stairs one step at a time?

13. Does your child seem very bright and articulate when in conversation but cannot seem to understand what he/she reads?

14. Is your child the class clown?

15. Is your child not working up to his/her potential?

16. Does your child seem to "tune-out" at times?

17. Is your child unusually forgetful?

18. Does your child find it necessary to touch everything he/she sees?

19. Does your child frequently walk into things or trip?

20. Is there inconsistency in your child's performance? (one day performs a task well, the next day can't)

21. Does your child have a short attention span?

22. Does your child move his/her lips while reading or follow the line with his/her fingers?

23. Does your child get frequent headaches?

24. Is your child ever purposely destructive?

25. Does your child frustrate easily?

26. Is your child unusually sensitive to light, noise, touch, or certain clothing material?

27. Was your child a late walker?

28. Was your child a prolonged tiptoe walker?

29. Was your child's speech late or abnormal?

30. Is your child a bed-wetter?

31. Does your child have uncontrollable rage reactions?

32. Does your child complain of seeing things bigger or smaller than they are?

33. Is your child unable to keep up with the other children's activity levels?

34. Does your child have a poor appetite?

35. Does your child have a history of allergies?

36. Is your child irritable before and/or shortly after meals?

37. Does your child crave sweets?

38. Has your child experienced excessive weight loss or weight gain?

39. Does your child frequently go out of the lines when coloring?

40. Did your child have trouble learning how to tie and/or button and/or lace?

41. Was your child colicky?

42. Was your child an unusually cranky baby?

43. Was your child an unusually passive baby?
44. Is your child a bully?
45. Is your child always picked on by his peers?
46. Is your child a loner?
47. Does your child seek out older or younger playmates?
48. Does your child's walking or running seem clumsy or disjointed?
49. When your child reads out loud, does he/she get mixed up or lose his/her place?
50. Does your child not complete his/her homework assignments?

High School
1. Does your child avoid sports or activities that involve catching or throwing a ball? or did he/she?
2. Does your child's walking or running seem uncoordinated or sloppy?
3. Is your child easily distractible?
4. Does your child confuse left from right?
5. Is/was your child always up and down from the table during meals?
6. Is your child a discipline problem?
7. Does your child seem very bright and articulate when in conversation but cannot seem to understand what he/she reads?
8. Is your child the class clown?
9. Is your child below grade level or not working to his/her potential?
10. Is your child unusually forgetful?
11. Does your child frequently walk into things or trip?
12. Is there inconsistency in your child's performance?
13. Does your child have a short attention span?
14. Does your child move his/her lips while reading or follow the lines with his/her fingers?
15. Does your child get frequent headaches?
16. Does your child frustrate easily?
17. Does your child have difficulty keeping rhythm while dancing or clapping?
18. Was your child a late walker?
19. Was your child a prolonged tiptoe walker?
20. Was your child's speech late or abnormal?
21. Does your child complain that words blur or move on the page?
22. Is your child always tired?
23. Does your child have a poor appetite?
24. Does your child have a history of anemia of any type?

25. Is your child irritable before and/or shortly after meals?

26. Does your child exhibit excessive thirst?

27. Does your child crave sweets?

28. Has your child experienced excessive weight gain or loss?

29. Did your child have trouble learning how to tie and/or button and/or lace?

30. Was your child colicky?

31. Was your child an unusually cranky baby?

32. Does/did your child have poor bowel or bladder control?

33. Does your child do everything to excess?

34. Is your child a bully?

35. Is your child always picked on by his/her peers?

36. Is your child a loner?

37. Does your child seek out older or younger playmates?

38. When your child reads out loud, does he/she get mixed up or lose his/her place?

39. Is your child ever purposely destructive?

40. Does your child fail to complete his or her homework assignments on time?

41. Is your child often truant from school?

42. Does it seem your child never pays attention to you?

43. Is your child unable to modulate his/her voice?

44. Does your child keep his/her head close to the paper or tilt it back and forth when reading or writing?

45. Does your child always seem to have a cold?

46. Does your child get frequent stomachaches?

47. Does your child seem to "tune-out" at times?

48. Does your child have uncontrollable rage reactions?

49. Does your child have a history of allergies?

50. Was your child an unusually passive baby?

CHAPTER 11

WILL YOU SURVIVE THE NEXT TEN YEARS? A HEALTH HAZARD APPRAISAL TEST

Given a large sampling of people of the same age, sex, and race, it is possible to predict how many of them will not survive a year, two years, or ten years. Conversely, it is possible to predict how many *will* survive. This information is contained in mortality tables published at regular intervals by the National Center for Health Statistics. Furthermore, it is possible to predict, with a fair degree of accuracy, how many in each group will die from specific causes: heart attack, stroke, motor vehicle accidents, the various cancers, pneumonia, suicide, homicide, and so on.

The statistics are presented per 100,000 people of a certain group. During the next ten years, for example, among any average group of 100,000 white males, age 40 to 44, 1,629 will die of the most common kind of heart disease, 348 will die of lung cancer, 275 will die in motor vehicle accidents. In all, 5,237 of these men will die for a variety of reasons.

Among 100,000 white females, age 40 to 44, only 348 may be expected to die of the same heart disease during the next ten years, 149 of lung cancer, and 93 in motor vehicle accidents. In all, 2,872 of these women will die from various causes.

As interest in preventive medicine grew during the last twenty to thirty years, doctors began to examine figures like these very carefully to see what could be done to reduce death and disability in some of the high-risk categories. One fact was obvious from the outset: although there are roughly one thousand causes of death, between one-half and three-quarters of the deaths in any population group can be attributed to ten or fifteen identifiable causes. If we can intervene in these top ten or fifteen causes, they reasoned, we can save many lives and prevent a great deal of disability.

Carrying this thinking a step further and refining the statistics to include health data developed over the past thirty years, it becomes apparent that some people in each of the population groups stand more of a chance than others of being among those who die or are disabled. These are termed high-risk people. A person who smokes, gets no exercise, is overweight, and has high blood pressure is at high risk from heart attack. Smokers are at high risk from lung cancer.

By looking at your health history and asking you about your health habits, a doctor can tell you what your *prospects* are for surviving the next ten years. The doctor can't guarantee life or death, but your *chances*, as compared to others in your population group, can be assessed. If you are at high risk, especially from those health hazards that account for most of the deaths in your group, the doctor can tell you what to do to improve your prospects for staying alive.

The name "prospective medicine," then, was proposed for that practice of medicine that begins with a well person and uses prospective studies as a guide to extend his or her life expectancy. The object of prospective medicine is to provide patients with a survival advantage over those in the general population, a tactic, incidentally, which is neither exclusive nor original with this method of practicing medicine. "Exercise," says the American Heart Association, "and you will have a survival advantage over those who don't." The American Cancer Society exhorts us not to smoke and shows us statistics to prove that those who do not smoke have a distinct survival advantage over those who do. Prospective medicine consolidates the known ways of providing patients with survival advantages and systematizes them into a method that is a combination of a doctor's treatment and supervision, and patient cooperation and self-help.

The basic procedures of prospective medicine were outlined in 1970 in a publication by Dr. Lewis C. Robbins and Dr. Jack H. Hall, both of the Methodist Hospital of Indiana at Indianapolis. The key to prospective medicine is the Health Hazard Appraisal in which a careful patient history is used to assess the distinct health risks of each patient. Once the risks are known, doctor and patient can intervene to reduce them, thereby producing a survival advantage for the patient. But it was recognized from the outset that setting a limited goal was best—a ten-year survival was chosen—and that the highest degree of cooperation between doctor and patient was crucial. Reducing the risks from most health hazards, in fact, depends entirely on the patient. Such procedures, for instance, as cutting down on alcohol consumption and not smoking can dramatically reduce your risk from six of the top fourteen causes of death. Weight control, getting adequate exercise, following orders for controlling blood pressure or diabetes are all areas where the doctor may propose but the patient must dispose if the program is to work.

Getting this kind of cooperation from a patient is not easy. The doctor uses the Health Hazard Appraisal, therefore, to demonstrate graphically what a person's risks are in relation to a large population of people of the same age and sex. At the end of the test the doctor can say, "Here are your risks of dying from certain specified causes during the next ten years, and here is your risk of dying from all causes compared with other average people like you." If your risks are high, the doctor can demonstrate that your health age is older than your chronological age. For example, a forty-year-old man with high risks may prove to be forty-five or fifty when his physical condition, health habits, and survival chances are considered. Such a demonstration is often enough to prompt compliance with a program designed to improve the risks and produce a survival advantage. Risks are reducible and effects are reversible.

The doctor can go on to show that the same forty-year-old man can take steps to improve his survival advantage to the point where his health age is actually younger than his chronological age. It is drama at its highest—hard to believe, but entirely true.

Specialists in family medicine, health-maintenance organizations, community-health clinics, and clinics at teaching hospitals are the most likely places to find some form of prospective medicine being practiced. But, for a variety of reasons, not all doctors think or practice in terms of appraising a patient's chances for ten-year survival. Prospective medicine as a system of health evaluation is only twenty years old; it is still rather new to a large part of the medical community. The Health Hazard Appraisal takes time and many doctors have neither the time nor the staff to handle it. Most medical practice is still crisis-oriented, dealing with patients who arrive sick, which is a sufficient load for a busy doctor; after all, the sick must still be cared for even as we try to think about keeping well people well.

As the present interest in preventive medicine continues to grow, however, you can expect to find more and more doctors practicing some form of prospective medicine. In the meantime, there is no reason why you can't do a Health Hazard Appraisal yourself, assess your present risks and take steps to reduce them.

SOME PREMISES OF THE TEST

The Health Hazard Appraisal is done twice. The first time you assess your present risks and the second time you see what your risks can be if you begin to monitor and manage your health—take steps to bring your weight under control, reduce your blood pressure, exercise, stop smoking, and so on. If you are not presently caring for your health, you will find the results amazing and perhaps a bit frightening.

The Health Hazard Appraisal used here is adapted from The Robbins and Hall instructional handbook, *How to Practice Prospective Medicine,*[1] and simplified for home use. Mortality statistics are based on the Geller-Steele "Tables of Dying in the Next Ten Years from Specific Causes."[2]

You will be comparing yourself with a population sampling of 100,000 people in the United States of the same sex and approximately the same age as you are. You will find that leading causes of death and the number of deaths from each cause vary considerably among different age groups and between males and females of the same age. Motor vehicle accidents, for instance, are the leading cause of death among people under thirty, and many more men than women die in accidents. Women, on the other hand, are at high risk from cancers of the breast, cervix, and uterus, while men, of course, are not.

In the Geller-Steele tables, and in the mortality tables of the National Center for Health Statistics, from which the Geller-Steele tables are derived, populations are also divided by race—white and black— because the leading causes of death are different for white people and black people of the same age and sex. The incidence of high blood pressure is much greater among blacks than among whites, for example, which greatly increases the risk of heart attack and stroke among black people. The death rate from many causes, in fact, is higher among black people. This higher mortality rate is heavily influenced by socio-economic factors and readers of all races should be aware that social and economic ills and injustices are of themselves distinct health hazards that work to shorten life.

The Health Hazard Appraisal we use here includes the ten causes of death for men and twelve for women which account for at least one-half of all deaths in any age group, and all the other causes of death combined will not change the statistics very much. Further, the risks dealt with here are reversible for the most part; that is, you can do something to reduce them.

The Health Hazard Appraisal assumes an "average" individual who is apparently well at the time the test is taken. If you have a serious

[1]Lewis C. Robbins, and Jack H. Hall, *How to Practice Prospective Medicine,* copyright 1970, Methodist Hospital of Indiana, Indianapolis.

[2]Harvey Geller and Gregory Steele, *Probability of Dying in the Next Ten Years from Specific Causes,* copyright pending, Methodist Hospital of Indiana.

chronic disease, or if you work at a particularly hazardous occupation, you can expect to be at higher risk than most people, and this is not reflected in the test.

You can do your calculations for the test directly in the book, or do them on a separate piece of paper if you want a copy of your figures for your personal health file. The arithmetic is rather easy—at about a fifth- or sixth-grade level—requiring only simple addition, subtraction, and multiplication, and knowing where to put the decimal point when you multiply decimals (example: $1.5 \times .2 = .30$).

Some of the information you need for the questionnaire must come from your doctor—your cholesterol level, for instance. Some information may come either from your doctor or from self-testing—your blood pressure and weight are among these. But much of the information required deals with your personal history and habits—your smoking, drinking, driving, and so on. Be honest. There is nothing to be gained from artificially reducing your risk factors except a false sense of security.

You will be led slowly through the first risk category, heart attack. Use the instructions found here to complete all of the categories.

HEALTH HAZARD APPRAISAL

Finding Your Risk Factors

HEART ATTACK

By the time a man reaches thirty-five, heart attack has become the number-one cause of death in his age group, so this is his greatest health risk. For women of the same age it is the number-two killer, running a close second behind breast cancer. Heart attack doesn't achieve the prominence of number one among women until age forty-five. By completing the following questionnaire and doing the simple arithmetic called for, you can assess your risk of dying of a heart attack during the next ten years as compared to the average population of people of your age and sex.

You will see what your *risk factor* is in several categories, and then putting them together you will find your total or *composite risk factor* for heart attack. At the end of the test we will use all of the composite risk factors to determine your *health age* as distinct from your chronological age. You may be older or younger than you think, as far as your statistical life expectancy is concerned.

As you complete the Health Hazard Appraisal it will quickly become apparent what you can do to reduce your risks and increase your statistical life expectancy. This is the whole point in doing the test twice—to see what the situation is and then what it can be if you start taking better care of yourself.

Look at the Health Hazard Appraisal for Heart Attack and follow these instructions:

1. In each category, select the risk factor that applies to you. If your risks seem to fall between the factors given, use an average of the two nearest risk factors that seem to apply to you.
2. If your risk factor is *1.0 or less,* enter it in the "×" column. If your risk factor is *more than 1.0,* enter it in the "+" column.
3. *Multiply* all of the figures you have entered in the "×" column together. If you have no figures in the "×" column, put in a 1.0 anyhow and that is your "×" column score.

    Add all the figures in the "+" column. *Subtract* from this total the *number of figures* you added. The result is the "+" column score.
4. Add the "×" score and the "+" score to get your composite risk factor for heart attack.

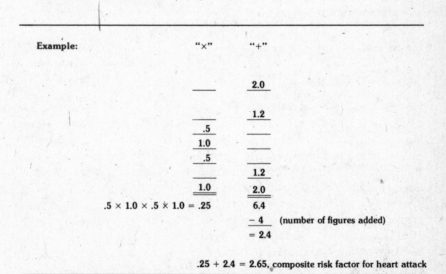

This would mean that your risk of dying of a heart attack during the next ten years is 2.65 times as great as an average person in your population group—those of the same age, sex and race as you are. Average is 1.0. If your composite risk factor is less than 1.0, you are at less risk from heart attack than an average person in your population group.

Risk from Heart Attack	Risk Factor	"×" (risk factors of 1.0 or less)	"+" (risk factors of more than 1.0)
Systolic blood pressure			
200 or more	3.0	_____	_____
180	2.0		
160	1.5		
140 or less	.5		
Diastolic blood pressure			
106	3.4	_____	_____
100	1.8		
94	1.2		
90 or less	1.0		
Cholesterol level			
280	1.5	_____	_____
220	1.0		
180	.5		
Diabetes			
Yes—and I do nothing about it	3.0	_____	_____
Yes—but under control with doctor's care	2.5		
No diabetes	1.0		
Exercise			
Little or none	2.5	_____	_____
Some exercise	1.0		
Regular, vigorous exercise	.5		
Parents who died of heart attack before age 60			
Both	1.5	_____	_____
One	1.2		
Neither or not known	1.0		
Smoking (choose highest which applies)			
Cigarettes	2.0	_____	_____
Cigars or pipe	1.0		
Nonsmoker	.5		
Weight			
75% overweight	2.5	_____	_____
50% overweight	1.5		
15% overweight	1.0		
10% underweight	.5		

$$\underline{\underline{}} \qquad \underline{\underline{}}$$

$$-\underline{} \text{ (number of figures)}$$

$$+\underline{}$$

$$=\underline{} \text{ , composite risk factor.}$$

STROKE

Stroke and heart attack both result from problems in the circulatory system, so you will find many of the same risk factors for both diseases. Find your composite risk factor the same way as you did for heart attack.

Risk from Stroke	Risk Factor	"×" (risk factors of 1.0 or less)	"+" (risk factors of more than 1.0)
Systolic blood pressure			
200 or more	3.0	_____	_____
180	2.3		
160	1.5		
140	1.0		
120 or less	.5		
Diastolic blood pressure			
106	3.8	_____	
100	2.2		
94	1.3		
88	.5		
Cholesterol level			
280	1.8	_____	_____
220	1.0		
180	.5		
Diabetes			
Yes—and I do nothing about it	3.0	_____	_____
Yes—but under control with doctor's care	2.5		
No diabetes	1.0		
Smoking (choose highest which applies)			
Cigarettes	1.5	_____	_____
Cigars or pipe	1.0		
Nonsmoker	.5		

$-$ _____ (number of figures)

_____ $+$ _____

$=$ _____ , composite risk factor.

MOTOR VEHICLE ACCIDENTS

Motor vehicle accidents are not usually thought of as a health hazard, but there's no good reason why they shouldn't be. No disease kills you more dead, no epidemic is as widespread or causes more disability. From age five to age thirty among men, and from five to twenty-five among women, motor vehicle accidents are the leading cause of death. More young children are lost to motor vehicle accidents than to any disease an anxious mother may worry about; and even men in their forties need to worry more about dying in an automobile than they need to worry about pneumonia or cancers of the digestive system.

Robbins and Hall have identified three major factors that affect your risk of dying in an automobile accident: alcohol habits, the mileage you travel by auto in a year, and whether or not you use seat belts. To this we have added speed. When the fifty-five miles per hour speed limit was imposed following the first oil crisis in 1973, and people were observing it, traffic fatalities plummeted. As we began ignoring this lower speed limit in subsequent years, auto fatalities began their inexorable rise once again.

When you assess your risk from motor vehicle accidents in the Health Hazard Appraisal, you must think of the driver when you are a passenger as well as the times when you drive yourself. Often, you are at greater risk as a passenger than as a driver.

Follow the same instructions for determining your composite risk factor for motor vehicle accidents as you did for heart attack and stroke.

Risk from Motor Vehicle Accidents	Risk Factor	"×" (risk factors of 1.0 or less)	"+" (risk factors of more than 1.0)
Alcohol habits			
Frequently excessive	5.0	_____	_____
Sometimes excessive	2.0		
Moderate social and home	1.0		
Nondrinker	.5		
Often use drugs and drive	2.0		
Mileage per year			
Divide miles traveled per year by 10,000. This is your risk factor. Include mileage driven with others.	_____	_____	_____
Seat belt use			
Less than 25% of the time	1.1	_____	_____
About 25% to 75%	1.0		
Most of the time	.8		
Speed habits			
Usually exceed posted limits	2.0	_____	_____
Sometimes exceed posted limits	1.0		
Rarely exceed posted limits	.5		

$$- \underline{\hspace{2cm}} \text{ (number of figures)}$$

$$+ \underline{\hspace{2cm}}$$

$$= \underline{\hspace{2cm}} , \text{composite risk factor.}$$

LUNG CANCER AND EMPHYSEMA

Despite pronouncements by the tobacco industry to the contrary, cigarette smoking greatly increases the risk from lung cancer and emphysema. It is true that other environmental pollutants besides cigarettes also contribute to the risk, and it is also true that some people smoke all their lives and live to be ninety. But *overwhelming* statistical evidence accumulated for more than thirty years demonstrates beyond doubt that cigarette smoking puts you at higher risk from lung cancer and emphysema.

Because you only select one risk factor for each of these diseases, based on your smoking habits, this is the same as your composite risk factor in each case. You don't have to do any further arithmetic this time.

Risk from Lung Cancer	Risk Factor	"×" (risk factors of 1.0 or less)	"+" (risk factors of more than 1.0)
Smoking habits			
Choose only *one* factor—the highest that applies to you:			
Cigarettes (daily average)			
Two packs	2.8		
One pack	2.0		
Half a pack	1.5		
Less than half a pack	.8		
		_____	_____
Cigars and pipe			
Over 5, or any inhaled	1.0		
Under 5, not inhaled	.5		
Nonsmoker	.5		
Former smoker			
One year—risk factor is 30% below risk while smoking.			
Two years or more—reduce risk an added 10% per year to a minimum .5.			
		Composite risk factor is the same as the one risk factor you chose: _____	

Risk from Emphysema			
Same risk factor as lung cancer, except if you are an exsmoker your present risk factor is 30% of what it would be if you still smoked as you once did.		_____	_____
Exsmokers: Calculate your risk as if you still smoked and multiply it by .3. Enter this figure.		Composite risk factor is the same as the one risk factor you chose: _____	

CANCER OF THE LARGE INTESTINE AND RECTUM

For some unknown, but fortunate reason, cancer of the stomach has been in a steady decline and at present, accounts for less than one percent of deaths even in the highest risk groups. Thus, it is not included in the Health Hazard Appraisal except under "other causes of death." Cancer of the small intestine is rather rare and is not included either. Cancer of the large intestine (colon) and of the rectum are still important threats, however, from about age thirty-five on.

Undiagnosed bleeding from the rectum puts you at higher risk of death from these cancers. It can appear as bright red blood or as black, tarry stools which indicates bleeding higher up in the digestive tract. You may reduce the risk factor on the Health Hazard Appraisal, however, if a doctor determines that the bleeding is harmless, or if the ailment causing the bleeding is otherwise diagnosed and you put yourself under the care and watchful eye of a physician. In any case, having an annual examination of the rectum and colon reduces your composite risk factor by two-thirds, as you will see. Examination doesn't prevent cancer, of course, but early discovery and prompt treatment increases your chance of survival if it does occur.

Ulcerative colitis increases your risk and should be given special attention by a doctor. Polyps, benign tumors that sometimes form in the large intestine, are also considered to put you at higher risk, not because they are dangerous in themselves, but because they have a reputation for turning bad. For this reason, many doctors advise removing them when they are discovered—a very simple procedure.

Figure your composite risk factor following the instructions given for heart attack.

Cancer of the Large Intestine and Rectum	Risk Factor	"×" (risk factors of 1.0 or less)	"+" (risk factors of more than 1.0)
Polyps			
Have had	2.5	_____	_____
Have not had	1.0		
Rectal bleeding, not diagnosed by a doctor			
Have had	3.0	_____	_____
Have not had	1.0		
Ulcerative colitis			
Have had ten years or more	4.0	_____	_____
Have had less than ten years	2.0		
Have not had	1.0		

$$-\underline{\qquad}\text{ (number of figures)}$$

$$\underline{\qquad} + \underline{\qquad}$$

$$=\underline{\qquad}\text{ , composite risk factor.*}$$

*If you have a regular annual examination of the rectum and colon by a physician, multiply the composite risk factor by 0.3 and use the lower figure.

SUICIDE AND HOMICIDE

These are two more risks we don't often think of as health hazards, but they most certainly are. Both ailments occur in epidemic proportions that far exceed the polio events that terrorized people in the 1930s and 1940s.

Suicide is a very mysterious phenomenon when it comes to determining who will or who won't destroy themselves. Two things seem fairly clear, however: there is a higher risk of suicide when mental depression is present, and risk is greater in families where there has been suicide before. Therefore, these two risks are included in the Health Hazard Appraisal. Keep in mind that the risks indicated are quite low, and the number of deaths from suicide, which we will present later, are quite understated. This is because for religious and social reasons families find a considerable onus attached to suicide, and to spare the feelings of bereaved families, doctors and investigating authorities frequently classify suicides as accidental death—falls, auto accidents, accidental drug poisoning, and so on.

Exposure to the risk of homicide takes many forms: living in a violent neighborhood, consorting with violence-prone individuals, having a violent nature yourself, engaging in criminal activity, excessive drinking in questionable surroundings. But there are two factors that are outstanding for increasing the risk of homicide: participating in violent crime and carrying a weapon. So these are the two indicators of risk used in the Health Hazard Appraisal.

Something to think about: 70 percent of deaths among boys fifteen to nineteen are caused by motor vehicle accidents, suicide, homicide, and other violent accidents. The rate among youths in their late twenties is not much better—about 60 percent violent deaths. Most of them are preventable.

Risk from Suicide	Risk Factor	"×" (risk factors of 1.0 or less)	"+" (risk factors of more than 1.0)
Depression			
Often depressed	2.5	_____	_____
Seldom or never	1.0		
Family history of suicide			
Yes	2.5	_____	_____
No	1.0		

– _____ (number of figures)

_____ + _____

= _____ , composite risk factor.

Risk from Homicide	Risk Factor	"×" (risk factors of 1.0 or less)	"+" (risk factors of more than 1.0)
Arrest record			
Crime including violence	10.0	_____	_____
Arrest for nonviolent crime	1.0		
Weapons			
Carry knife or gun	2.0	_____	_____
Do not carry	1.0		

– _____ (number of figures)

_____ + _____

= _____ , composite risk factor.

CIRRHOSIS OF THE LIVER AND PNEUMONIA

In cirrhosis, the liver is damaged and becomes scarred to the point where blood cannot flow through it properly and its function is badly impaired. Symptoms sometimes go unnoticed until the disease has made considerable progress toward destroying the liver. While it's possible to treat cirrhosis and impede its progress, liver tissue that has been destroyed cannot be restored. If the disease is allowed to go unchecked, blood that cannot flow through the liver may back up into the esophagus until blood vessels there rupture and there is severe internal bleeding.

There are several causes of liver damage but the prime cause in our society is too much alcohol. Therefore, only one risk is included in the Health Hazard Appraisal, which is related to the way you use alcohol. The risk factor that applies is also the composite risk factor for cirrhosis.

Since the discovery of penicillin, pneumonia is not the dread disease it once was, but it is still dreadful enough to account for between 2 percent and 4 percent of deaths in most age groups. Of the people who die there are more among heavy drinkers, cigarette smokers, those with emphysema, and those who have had pneumonia before in either its viral or bacterial forms. Because there are several risk factors to consider here, you will figure your composite risk factor in the usual way.

Risk from Cirrhosis of the Liver	Risk Factor	"×" (risk factors of 1.0 or less)	"+" (risk factors of more than 1.0)
Alcohol habits			
Alcoholic	12.5	_____	_____
Frequently excessive	5.0		
Sometimes excessive	2.0		
Usually moderate	1.0		
Infrequent or nondrinker	.2		

Composite risk factor is the same as the one risk factor you chose: _____

Risk from Pneumonia	Risk Factor	"×" (risk factors of 1.0 or less)	"+" (risk factors of more than 1.0)
Alcohol habits			
Often excessive	3.0	_____	_____
Moderate or nondrinker	1.0		
Had pneumonia before			
Yes	2.0	_____	_____
No	1.0		
Emphysema			
Have emphysema	2.0	_____	_____
Do not have	1.0		
Smoking habits			
Cigarette smoker	1.2	_____	_____
Other smokers and nonsmokers	1.0		

−_____ (number of figures)

_____ + _____

=_____ , composite risk factor.

CANCER OF THE BREAST, CERVIX, AND UTERUS

Not too long ago, the diagnosis of these cancers was equivalent to a death sentence, usually because discovery was made late in the course of the disease. The picture has changed, however. Women are encouraged to regularly avail themselves of the two techniques that uncover breast and uterine cancer in their early stages: the Pap smear for early detection of uterine cancer and breast self-examination for early detection of breast cancer.

More breast cancers are discovered by women themselves than by doctors, and it is estimated that as many as 75,000 women a year are saved by the Pap smear. More than one doctor has said that it is beyond understanding why Doctor Papanicolau, who devised the test and for whom it is named, was never awarded a Nobel prize for his work.

While breast cancer is not inherited, it seems to occur more frequently in families where it has occurred before. It happens enough times so that this is considered to put a woman at somewhat higher risk for the purposes of Health Hazard Appraisal. But regular self-examination seems to return these women to the average risk of the general population. Self-examination does not prevent breast cancer, of course, but early detection resulting from self-examination does save lives when treatment is promptly begun.

Vaginal bleeding that is not related to menstrual periods and that has not been diagnosed by a gynecologist puts you at higher risk from uterine cancer. Once the cause has been diagnosed as noncancerous and is treated, you may be considered at average risk once again.

As everyone knows, most of the causes of cancer are as elusive of scientific investigation as are the cures. But statistical observations point to one group or another who are more susceptible or less susceptible to certain cancers than other groups for reasons that are not entirely understood. Where cancer of the cervix is concerned, Jewish women seem to be at very low risk. Social and economic status also seem to play a part, with women in low economic groups more susceptible than their more fortunate sisters. And early onset of intercourse seems to increase the risk of cervical cancer over women who begin later.

Since you select only one risk factor for breast cancer, this is also your composite risk factor. There is more than one risk factor for cancer of the cervix and uterus, so figure your composite risk factor here in the usual way. Because the Pap smear is so important, you can reduce your composite risk factor, as shown, if you have been having it done.

Risk from Breast Cancer	Risk Factor	"×" (risk factors of 1.0 or less)	"+" (risk factors of more than 1.0)
Mother or sister had breast cancer			
Yes	2.0	_____	_____
Yes, but I do a regular self-exam	1.0		
No	1.0		
Neither had breast cancer *and* I do regular self-exam	.5		

Composite risk factor is the same as the one risk factor you chose: _____

Risk from Cancer of the Cervix and Uterus			
Vaginal bleeding, undiagnosed			
Yes, have had	2.0	_____	_____
Have not had	1.0		
Economic and social status			
Low	2.0	_____	_____
Average	1.0		
High	.5		
Jewish			
No	1.0	_____	_____
Yes	.1		
Onset of intercourse			
Teenage	2.5	_____	_____
20–25	1.0		
Over 25	.7		

‑ _____ (number of figures)

_____ + _____

= _____ composite risk factor.*

*If you have had Pap smears as indicated, multiply your composite risk by the appropriate number and use the new, lower score:

   1 negative within 5 years .7
   1 negative within 1 year   .5
   3 negative within 5 years .1

YOUR HEALTH APPRAISAL AGE: ARE YOU OLDER OR YOUNGER THAN YOUR LAST BIRTHDAY AGE?

Your Present Risk and What It Can Be.   As you filled in your risk factors it had to be very clear to you what you are doing wrong and what you are doing right where your health is concerned. If your composite risk factors are consistently less than 1.0, it means you are living the good life (a healthy life) and, statistically speaking, your chances for surviving the next ten years are considerably better than most people in your population group—people of the same age, sex, and race as you are.

Where your risk factors are more than 1.0, your risk from that disease is higher than an average person in your group. A composite score of 2.5 for heart attack means that statistically you are two and one-half times more likely to suffer a fatal heart attack in the next ten years than the average person in your group.

These are statistics, of course, and they do not guarantee that any one individual *will not* die of a heart attack because his or her risk factors are low, or that someone else *will* die of a heart attack because his or her risk factors are high. The point is this: A certain limited number of people who are presently the same age and sex as you are will die of heart attacks during the next ten years. If someone has to bet money that you will not be among the heart-attack fatalities ten years from now, his money will be safer if your risk factors are low.

But as we have said before, many risks are reversible. If your risk from heart attack is high because you smoke, are overweight, and have high blood pressure, you can reduce the odds tremendously if you quit smoking, lose weight, and have the doctor treat your high blood pressure.

Do the Health Hazard Appraisal a second time, this time assuming that you will change your health habits and do everything right. See what your new risk factors can be if you take care of yourself.

Filling Out the Health Hazard Appraisal Chart.   We will now go on to see what the risk factors mean in terms of numbers of people who may be expected to die in the next ten years in your population group of 100,000. This will lead to a determination of whether you are younger or older than you think you are—your Health Appraisal Age. To do this you must fill out the Health Hazard Appraisal Chart. Follow these instructions:

1. In column 1, next to each disease listed, enter the number of average people per 100,000 of your age, sex, and race who are

expected to die from the disease during the next ten years. You can get this information from the tables in the following pages. Use Table 1 if you are white and Table 2 if you are black.

2. In column 2, enter your *composite risk factor* for each disease, which you found by doing your Health Hazard Appraisal. The last item is "All Other Causes." Use 1.0 as your risk factor here.

3. Multiply the number of deaths by your composite risk factor for each disease. This tells you how many people per 100,000 *with your level of risk* may be expected to die during the next ten years from each disease listed. This is your present risk from each health hazard.

4. Add column 3. This gives you your *total personal risk* which you will use to find your Health Appraisal Age.

5. Now, find this total down one side of Table 3 if you are white, Table 4 if you are black. These are the Health Age Tables. One side is for males, the other for females.

6. To find your Health Age, go down the column that is headed with the *last digit* of your actual age: 2, if you are 42; 9, if you are 29; 0, if you are 50, and so on. (Notice that each column is headed with *two* last digits to save space.) The age in this column across from the closest number to your total personal risk is your *Health Appraisal Age*. Compare this with your actual age on your nearest birthday.

HEALTH HAZARD APPRAISAL CHART

Disease	(1) Number of deaths from Table 1 or 2		(2) Your composite risk factor		(3) Columns (1) × (2) = your present risk
Heart attack		×		=	
Stroke		×		=	
Motor vehicle accidents		×		=	
Lung cancer		×		=	
Emphysema		×		=	
Cancer of colon and rectum		×		=	
Suicide		×		=	
Homicide		×		=	
Cirrhosis of the liver		×		=	
Pneumonia		×		=	
Breast cancer		×		=	
Cancer of cervix and uterus		×		=	
All other causes		×	1.0	=	

(Your total
personal risk)

TABLE 1

Probable Deaths per 100,000 Population from Various Causes in Ten Years[1]

WHITES M = Male F = Female	Heart Attack	Stroke	Motor Vehicle Accidents	Lung Cancer	Emphysema	Cancer, Large Intestine and Rectum	Suicide	Homicide	Cirrhosis of the Liver	Pneumonia	Breast Cancer	Cancer of Cervix and Uterus	All Other Causes	Total Deaths
M 20–24	17	19	581	3	3	4	250	164	11	19	–	–	694	1765
F 20–24	5	20	139	2	2	4	77	45	7	15	10	8	316	650
M 25–29	71	28	403	11	4	12	240	163	38	21	–	–	780	1771
F 25–29	19	31	103	7	3	9	91	66	19	18	38	15	391	810
M 30–34	254	56	325	46	7	25	244	159	98	31	–	–	903	2148
F 30–34	54	60	90	24	6	22	105	46	49	24	97	29	564	1170
M 35–39	723	106	290	141	15	44	250	148	200	49	–	–	1234	3200
F 35–39	136	108	91	66	10	46	125	*	101	35	186	61	844	1809
M 40–44	1629	178	275	348	38	86	260	128	343	75	–	–	1877	5237
F 40–44	308	174	93	149	20	87	143	*	170	52	342	94	1240	2872
M 45–49	2973	299	260	681	88	172	281	109	471	113	–	–	2851	8298
F 45–49	624	268	92	249	47	161	145	*	232	74	518	131	1787	4328
M 50–54	5001	541	248	1188	198	314	301	*	580	191	–	–	4705	13267
F 50–54	1260	422	80	386	94	277	131	*	284	99	684	164	2686	6567
M 55–59	7809	979	258	1888	411	530	307	*	667	312	–	–	7533	20694
F 55–59	2406	699	*	517	148	434	*	*	311	148	807	180	4171	9821
M 60–64	11273	1775	258	2561	736	814	289	*	693	483	–	–	11601	30483
F 60–64	4307	1241	*	501	208	631	*	*	290	231	859	202	5941	14411
M 65–69	15622	3218	*	2998	1152	1121	*	*	615	785	–	–	18439	43950
F 65–69	7755	2464	*	500	264	900	*	*	245	383	921	269	8747	22448
M 70–74	21374	5583	*	3176	1552	1464	*	*	*	1431	–	–	28856	63436
F 70–74	13666	5070	*	564	314	1232	*	*	*	777	1018	299	14254	37203
M 75–79	27265	8581	*	2796	1677	1730	*	*	*	2386	–	–	21920	66355
F 75–79	21274	8815	*	512	327	1533	*	*	*	1467	1056	*	15369	50353

* Included with other causes. Omit from your Health Hazard Appraisal Chart.

[1]From Geller-Steele "Tables of Dying in the Next Ten Years from Specific Causes," Probability of Dying in the Next Ten Years from Specific Causes, copyright pending 1977, Methodist Hospital of Indiana.

TABLE 2
Probable Deaths per 100,000 Population from Various Causes in Ten Years[1]

BLACKS M = Male F = Female	Heart Attack	Stroke	Motor Vehicle Accidents	Lung Cancer	Emphysema	Cancer, Large Intestine and Rectum	Suicide	Homicide	Cirrhosis of the Liver	Pneumonia	Breast Cancer	Cancer of Cervix and Uterus	All Other Causes	Total Deaths
M 20–24	47	47	521	3	*	17	216	1596	58	52	–	–	1695	4252
F	19	47	112	*	*	9	48	313	38	31	14	18	823	1472
M 25–29	159	102	472	16	*	22	223	1617	215	97	–	–	2025	4948
F	76	96	106	6	*	14	54	300	122	51	49	49	1026	1949
M 30–34	415	197	431	82	27	27	184	1501	448	177	–	–	2545	6034
F	200	187	104	24	*	31	*	288	241	82	136	108	1491	2892
M 35–39	977	384	422	254	46	55	153	1340	651	249	–	–	3441	7972
F	490	358	99	82	*	59	*	259	351	111	251	165	2112	4337
M 40–44	2034	677	393	607	56	104	*	1110	834	322	–	–	4856	10993
F	1061	597	93	194	*	96	*	196	468	143	404	213	2967	6432
M 45–49	3476	1029	391	1183	101	184	*	987	919	416	–	–	7643	15259
F	1834	893	87	311	*	172	*	162	486	180	584	286	4080	9075
M 50–54	5332	1583	410	1893	192	288	*	806	878	533	–	–	9639	21154
F	3042	1348	*	421	*	316	*	*	458	207	703	402	5855	12752
M 55–59	7608	2400	396	2437	294	487	*	612	783	683	–	–	12531	28231
F	4697	2007	*	487	*	491	*	*	402	258	730	522	7726	17320
M 60–64	10138	3514	370	2709	429	716	*	461	621	856	–	–	16100	35914
F	6782	3032	*	458	*	638	*	*	276	369	748	571	9890	22764
M 65–69	14229	5367	406	2958	550	971	*	335	436	971	–	–	22795	49088
F	11110	5210	*	465	*	946	*	*	*	653	826	716	15514	35440
M 70–74	18323	7382	395	2834	607	1282	*	*	*	1677	–	–	31064	63564
F	15157	7485	*	480	*	1133	*	*	*	936	812	773	20752	47528
M 75–79	20641	8657	325	2273	606	1348	*	*	*	2212	–	–	35552	71614
F	17774	9121	*	416	*	1101	*	*	*	1184	722	664	22579	53561

* Included with other causes. Omit from your Health Hazard Appraisal Chart.

[1]From Geller-Steele "Tables of Dying in the Next Ten Years from Specific Causes."

TABLE 3
Your Health Age

Use the column headed by the last digit of your actual age

WHITE MALE Find number closest to your total personal risk	0 / 5	1 / 6	2 / 7	3 / 8	4 / 9
1760	15	16	17	18	19
1761	16	17	18	19	20
1762	17	18	19	20	21
1763	18	19	20	21	22
1764	19	20	21	22	23
1765	20	21	22	23	24
1766	21	22	23	24	25
1767	22	23	24	25	26
1768	23	24	25	26	27
1769	24	25	26	27	28
1771	25	26	27	28	29
1842	26	27	28	29	30
1915	27	28	29	30	31
1992	28	29	30	31	32
2069	29	30	31	32	33
2148	30	31	32	33	34
2324	31	32	33	34	35
2514	32	33	34	35	36
2721	33	34	35	36	37
2944	34	35	36	37	38
3200	35	36	37	38	39
3526	36	37	38	39	40
3886	37	38	39	40	41
4282	38	39	40	41	42
4719	39	40	41	42	43
5237	40	41	42	43	44
5735	41	42	43	44	45
6279	42	43	44	45	46
6876	43	44	45	46	47
7529	44	45	46	47	48

WHITE FEMALE Find number closest to your total personal risk	WHITE MALE number (continued)	0 / 5	1 / 6	2 / 7	3 / 8	4 / 9	WHITE FEMALE number (continued)
590	8298	45	46	47	48	49	4328
601	9103	46	47	48	49	50	4700
614	9986	47	48	49	50	51	5104
626	10955	48	49	50	51	52	5543
639	12017	49	50	51	52	53	6020
650	13267	50	51	52	53	54	6567
679	14501	51	52	53	54	55	7119
709	15849	52	53	54	55	56	7716
742	17323	53	54	55	56	57	8365
775	18934	54	55	56	57	58	9067
810	20694	55	56	57	58	59	9821
872	22350	56	57	58	59	60	10607
940	24137	57	58	59	60	61	11455
1012	26068	58	59	60	61	62	12372
1090	28154	59	60	61	62	63	13361
1170	30483	60	61	62	63	64	14411
1275	32769	61	62	63	64	65	15737
1390	35227	62	63	64	65	66	17185
1515	37869	63	64	65	66	67	18766
1652	40709	64	65	66	67	68	20492
1809	43950	65	66	67	68	69	22448
1981	47290	66	67	68	69	70	24828
2169	50884	67	68	69	70	71	27459
2375	54751	68	69	70	71	72	30370
2601	58913	69	70	71	72	73	33589
2872	63436	70	71	72	73	74	37203
3116							
3381							
3668							
3980							

TABLE 4
Your Health Age

Use the column headed by the last digit of your actual age

BLACK MALE Find number closest to your total personal risk	0 / 5	1 / 6	2 / 7	3 / 8	4 / 9	BLACK FEMALE Find number closest to your total personal risk
2851	15	16	17	18	19	1070
3088	16	17	18	19	20	1140
3344	17	18	19	20	21	1214
3621	18	19	20	21	22	1293
3922	19	20	21	22	23	1377
4252	20	21	22	23	24	1472
4384	21	22	23	24	25	1556
4520	22	23	24	25	26	1645
4660	23	24	25	26	27	1738
4804	24	25	26	27	28	1837
4948	25	26	27	28	29	1949
5146	26	27	28	29	30	2109
5352	27	28	29	30	31	2282
5566	28	29	30	31	32	2469
5788	29	30	31	32	33	2671
6034	30	31	32	33	34	2892
6378	31	32	33	34	35	3135
6742	32	33	34	35	36	3398
7126	33	34	35	36	37	3684
7532	34	35	36	37	38	3993
7972	35	36	37	38	39	4337
8498	36	37	38	39	40	4693
9059	37	38	39	40	41	5077
9657	38	39	40	41	42	5494
10294	39	40	41	42	43	5944
10993	40	41	42	43	44	6432
11730	41	42	43	44	45	6889
12515	42	43	44	45	46	7377
13354	43	44	45	46	47	7902
14249	44	45	46	47	48	8463

BLACK MALE number (continued)	0 / 5	1 / 6	2 / 7	3 / 8	4 / 9	BLACK FEMALE number (continued)
15259	45	46	47	48	49	9075
16281	46	47	48	49	50	9710
17372	47	48	49	50	51	10390
18536	48	49	50	51	52	11117
19778	49	50	51	52	53	11895
21154	50	51	52	53	54	12752
22402	51	52	53	54	55	13555
23724	52	53	54	55	56	14409
25124	53	54	55	56	57	15317
26606	54	55	56	57	58	16282
28231	55	56	57	58	59	17320
29614	56	57	58	59	60	18290
31065	57	58	59	60	61	19314
32588	58	59	60	61	62	20396
34184	59	60	61	62	63	21538
35914	60	61	62	63	64	22764
38213	61	62	63	64	65	24858
40658	62	63	64	65	66	27145
43260	63	64	65	66	67	29643
46029	64	65	66	67	68	32370
49088	65	66	67	68	69	35440
51690	66	67	68	69	70	37566
54429	67	68	69	70	71	39820
57314	68	69	70	71	72	42210
60352	69	70	71	72	73	44742
63564	70	71	72	73	74	47528

If you are older than you should be, refigure the totals in the Health Hazard Appraisal Chart using the composite risk factors that will apply once you change your health habits for the better. See what your Health Age *can be* if you look after yourself.

If your Health Age is younger than your actual age, congratulations! Keep up the good work. Continue to track your health and consult with a doctor as soon as you notice anything questionable.

There is one further thought you should keep in mind while you have your risk factors in front of you. The charts deal only with numbers of people who *die* as a result of various health hazards; many more people are disabled by the same diseases. Good health habits not only increase your chances for surviving, they increase your chances for a vital existence long after others your age have forgotten what good health is.

CHAPTER 12

CREATING A MEDICAL HISTORY AND PERSONAL HEALTH RECORD

Every medical testing program must begin with a comprehensive medical history, whether a doctor does it or you do it yourself. As you will see, there are many reasons why a well-kept personal record is a valuable health document and is usually superior to a patchwork of professional records scattered around the country among many doctors. It is the means by which you track the performance of your body systems and keep an eye on your health habits—and it plays no small role in keeping you well, in heading off serious illness, and in prolonging your life. In addition, a complete and documented personal health history is the most important diagnostic tool you can give to a doctor when you go to seek treatment.

Not long ago, a study was done in England to determine the relative values of a medical history, a physical examination, and laboratory tests in diagnosing a patient's condition. First, doctors at a general medical clinic were asked to diagnose their cases after they had done nothing more than take a careful medical history. They were asked again for the most likely diagnosis after they had done a physical examination, and again after they had the results of all the tests and X rays they had ordered.

In about 85 percent of the cases, the doctors made a correct diagnosis on the basis of the medical history alone! The physical examination increased the correct diagnosis rate by only 5 percent, and the medical tests by only 5 percent more. Finally, when all the data was available, no certain diagnosis could be made in the remaining 5 percent of patients.

The study concluded that the medical history gives doctors most of the information they need to make a correct diagnosis while examinations and tests serve to make the doctors' opinions more conclusive and supply the confidence needed to prescribe appropriate treatment.

WHAT IS A MEDICAL HISTORY?

A medical history may be created from the response to a single question such as "Well, now, what seems to be the trouble?" or it may be a complete record of everything medically significant in your life from the time you were born. It depends on what you and your doctor expect to accomplish together. If you are making a transient visit to the doctor with an injured thumb, or if you are seeking relief from what is obviously a head cold, neither you nor the doctor will want to spend a lot of time on the history of your life. But if your problem seems to be serious or puzzling, if you are seeking a complete appraisal of your health, or if you expect the doctor to supervise your health care for a number of years, there is much the doctor needs to know about you.

A typical history begins with a simple discussion of what may be troubling you at the moment. If you do have a complaint, the doctor will want you to describe your symptoms, how long you have had them, and how you noticed them developing. Then there is a probing of your past history, often a chronology from childhood until now. You will be asked about any chronic illnesses you may have, treatments you receive regularly, medicines you take, corrective devices you use.

Because some diseases are hereditary and others tend to run in families, the doctor will want to know about the health of your parents and grandparents, sisters and brothers. Then there is a long litany of questions that probes for information about allergies, diseases you have had, immunizations, operations, accidents, and injuries. There are personal questions: What do you do for a living and what do you do in your leisure time? Do you smoke, drink, diet? Are you satisfied with your life? with your sex life? Are you worried, unhappy or depressed?

You will be questioned about the functioning of all your body parts and systems, and you will be asked if you have noticed anything that seems unusual or has caused you concern. The more detailed and precise you can be about all this, the more the doctor has to work with when it comes to analyzing the state of your health.

HOW IS A LAY PERSON QUALIFIED
TO TAKE A MEDICAL HISTORY?

If you have ever filled out a medical questionnaire for an insurance company or as part of an application to participate in an athletic program, you probably recall that you supplied most of the information yourself while your doctor had only a few questions to answer based on a brief medical examination. In spite of the brief participation of a doctor, however, these questionnaires are quite reliable for health-screening purposes, and the reason they are reliable is that you are the world's leading expert on your own medical history. You are, in fact, the *only* person with a detailed knowledge of what has been happening to your body over the years; you know most about the family you were born into and you know most about the environment and social atmosphere in which your body must function.

Good doctors are expert at taking medical histories, but this simply means they have highly developed interviewing skills in the medical field rather than detailed knowledge of any one individual. Probing for special information in special situations, organizing and analyzing information and drawing medical conclusions—all of which require a physician's training and experience—come *after* you have supplied the bulk of the necessary medical history.

WHY YOU SHOULD KEEP A MEDICAL HISTORY AND PERSONAL HEALTH RECORD

There are several major weaknesses in medical histories taken in the doctor's office. First, considering the level of pressure in many busy medical offices, there isn't always time to search your memory for things that happened years ago. And memories are fallible; it just isn't possible to remember all of your past illnesses, treatments, and inoculations.

Many doctor-kept histories are taken when you are ill, because most people see a doctor only in times of sickness and distress. Histories taken at such times are full of bias and inaccuracies. Often, changes in your body and its functioning are more significant than signs, symptoms, and even test results at any one time on any one visit to a doctor's office. Increases in blood pressure, weight gain or loss, changing vision, changes in the texture of the breasts, changes in your skin, and changes in the operation of your digestive system are all of the utmost medical importance and they are all more apparent to you, if you have been tracking your health, than they are at any one time to an examining physician.

Our new consciousness of occupational dangers and environmental pollution has made many people wish they had begun keeping health records many years ago. Chemicals, industrial dirt and dust, radiation, drugs taken during pregnancy can all prove dangerous years after exposure to them. Without records, people often forget they have been exposed to these dangers or they are totally unaware that they have been exposed to a dangerous combination of elements. And without records to provide a clue, diagnosis of resulting ailments is often difficult and sometimes impossible.

Finally, we are a highly mobile society. Most people can recall treatment by a dozen or more doctors, often in medical facilities scattered across the country; and while medical records can be transferred from one doctor to another, few of us ever bother to have it done. It is a slow, tedious process, and if a medical emergency arises there is certainly no time to write or call around to gather essential facts.

Thousands of times every day, throughout the country, patients turn up at the emergency receiving room of a hospital where the first person they meet is a doctor who is an absolute stranger. This physician knows nothing about them, their medical difficulties, the state of their body systems, their allergies, or blood chemistry. Yet he or she must take immediate action. Under such circumstances diagnoses can be made more quickly and proper treatment prescribed more accurately when a medical history is available. Even in nonemergency medical situations, both time and money can be saved and medical treatment can be more satisfactory when the attending physician has a medical history and health record to work from.

HOW TO GET STARTED

Just the thought of assembling all the data that goes into a medical history may seem overwhelming at first, but it's not that difficult to do. You can set down most of the basic facts in an hour or so and then gather other information as it is convenient. It could be the most important bit of work you've ever done for yourself and your family. All the questions you need to answer for a complete medical history and health record can be found in the following pages. To get started, pick up a pencil and fill in the easiest things first: name, birthdate, place of birth, address, and phone number. Once begun, the information will seem to pour forth, begging to be recorded.

Writing a medical history and personal health record makes a fascinating and educational family project when parents and children work together. In addition to creating valuable health documents that will serve each family member for a lifetime, you will have an opportunity to teach children about their bodies, discuss health problems, sex and sexuality, and expose hidden fears that may not come to light otherwise.

When doing medical histories as a family project, each family member should have his or her own record.

There is no special way to proceed as long as you do a thorough job and furnish all the information you can. Here are some tips that will help:

1. Do what is easiest for you first, then go back and fill in information that may require a little digging in your memory or inquiries among other members of the family.

2. Some information may have to be obtained from a doctor: cholesterol level, blood type, blood pressure if you don't take it yourself, and so on. If you have had a recent physical examination, call the doctor's office and ask for the information you need. The office assistant can give it to you. If you haven't had a recent examination, this will give you a good excuse to do it now, and be sure to get all the information you need for your record from the doctor or the doctor's assistant at the time of your examination.

3. If you have moved or changed doctors and there are valuable records scattered about the country, write for them. Some hospitals and doctors may not want to send information directly to you, so arrange to have it sent to your local doctor. If you have lost the address of a doctor or other health facility, local libraries have telephone books from all over the country which you can use to find it. Libraries also have national directories of doctors and hospitals you can use. Ask the reference librarian in any medium-size library. State and county medical societies also have national directories and most of them will help you find the information you need.

4. You can get much of the information called for from self-testing. Watch for notes in the medical history that direct you to specific chapters of the *Bodyworkbook*.

5. Some information has to be updated regularly. Be sure to do this as often as indicated.

MEDICAL HISTORY AND PERSONAL HEALTH RECORD

Name _____ Phone (__) _____

Address _____

Occupation_____

Date of Birth_____ Birthplace _____

Blood Type _____ Rh factor _____ Race _____

(Blood type and Rh factor may be available from military records, Red Cross blood donor card, or employment records. If not, ask your doctor to check on your next visit.)

My body temperature when I am well varies

from _____ to _____
        oral
        rectal
        axillary (armpit).

(Check with a thermometer several times over a period of several days. Circle method used to measure temperature.)

CONTENTS OF MEDICAL HISTORY AND PERSONAL HEALTH RECORD

1. Family History
2. Immunization Record
3. Personal Health Habits
4. Weight-tracking
5. Occupational Health Hazards
6. Record of Physical Examinations by a Physician or Other Health Professional
7. Personal Illness Record
8. Operations
9. X ray Record
10. Tracking the Function of the Heart, Lungs, and Circulation
11. Tracking Vision
12. Tracking the Nervous System
13. Tracking Urine and the Urinary System
14. Tracking Digestive Function
15. Problems with Bones, Joints, and Muscles
16. Checking the Ears, Nose, Mouth, and Throat
17. Dental Record
18. Watching Your Skin
19. Problems with the Reproductive Organs
20. Other Concerns
21. A Systems Review

1. Family History

Some diseases are hereditary and others seem to run in families. Some diseases are more common among people of a particular race or from a certain part of the world.

In the following chart tell what you can about serious chronic illnesses and the causes of death among your closest *blood* relatives—not step- or adoptive relatives. The only nonblood relative you should include is a spouse since chronic illness in a husband or wife may provide important information about family life.

Begin with your father, mother, brothers, sisters, children, and spouse. Next, list blood-related aunts and uncles; omit cousins. Provide information about the diseases listed and any others that caused death or that you consider important.

Birth defects	Stroke	Liver disease
Cancer	Bleeding	Digestive tract ulcers
Leukemia	Anemia	Kidney disease
Tuberculosis	Epilepsy	Mental illness
Diabetes	Migraine headaches	Suicide
Heart trouble	Glaucoma	Alcoholism
Heart attack	Asthma	Drug addiction
High blood pressure	Emphysema	Allergies
		Others

Name and Relationship	Age if Living	Age at Death	Illness	Cause of Death	Comments

2. Immunization Record

Immunization records are often required for school, for certain jobs, and for foreign travel. Keep this record up-to-date and file any certificates in a place where they will be easy to find when needed.

Immunization is not just for young, preschool children. If you are uncertain about what inoculations you or your children have had (regardless of age), ask your physician to recommend a suitable procedure.

	Date	Date	Date	Date	Reactions or Side Effects, if Any
Diphtheria					
* Whooping cough					
Tetanus					
Polio					
* German measles					
Mumps					
** Smallpox					
Typhoid					
Others (Please list)					

*Often given together, but may be given separately.
**Smallpox is now said to be totally eradicated worldwide. Therefore, vaccination against smallpox is no longer required by many countries.

3. Personal Health Habits

A. Caffeine Consumption

Which of the following caffeine-containing beverages do you drink on a daily basis?

	Yes	No	6-oz. Servings Per Day
Coffee			
Tea			
Cola			

B. Smoking (Any Substance) and Drinking Alcohol

Do you smoke?_____ If yes, what do you smoke and how much? _____

_____

How would you describe your drinking habits?

_____ Alcoholic   _____ Usually moderate
_____ Frequently excessive   _____ Drink very little
_____ Sometimes excessive   _____ Nondrinker

C. Drugs and Medicines

List any drugs and medicines you use or have used frequently or for a long period of time.

	Name or Brand Name	How much?	When and for How Long?
Over-the-counter drugs*			
Prescription drugs** Illegal drugs			

*aspirin, laxatives, cold medications, etc.
**birth control, blood pressure, cortisone, antibiotics, tranquilizers, etc.

D. Special Diets

Are you on a special diet now or have you been in the recent past? If so, give dates, describe it, tell why you started the diet and the results.

Self-administered diet: _____

_____

_____

_____

_____

Prescribed special diet: _____

_____

_____

_____

_____

_____

E. Allergies

List substances you are allergic to (any food, penicillin, other drugs, cosmetics, fabrics, animals, plants, insect stings, etc.) and explain how you know you are allergic (adverse reactions, side effects). Describe any desensitizing treatments you have had. Do you have a bee-sting kit? Do you wear any kind of medical alert bracelet or necklace? _____

_____

_____

F. Emotional State

Answer the following questions "yes" or "no," and then make any comments or explanations in the space provided. If you feel it is not wise to write down answers that you do not want others in the family to see, just think about the questions and bring them up when you visit a physician or other counselor.

Do you find your life—
satisfactory _____   boring _____
unsatisfactory _____   too demanding _____

Comments and explanations: _____

_____

_____

_____

_____

_____

_____

_____

Do you worry about—

money _____	homelife _____
job _____	children _____
marriage _____	sex _____

Comments and explanations:_____
_____
_____
_____

Do you often—

cry easily_____	feel anxious or upset_____
feel inferior_____	feel nothing goes right___
feel worthless_____	feel depressed_____
feel shy_____	feel afraid for no reason
	_____

Comments and explanations: _____
_____
_____
_____

Have you—

seriously considered suicide _____ If so, when?_____
  attempted suicide _____ If so, when? _____

Comments and explanations:_____
_____
_____
_____

Do you have difficulty sleeping? _____ If yes, describe your sleep habits and patterns—when you go to bed, whether you take naps, whether you use tranquilizers or sleeping pills of any kind, how and where you sleep, etc.

_____
_____
_____

G. Tracking Periods of Depression

In the following chart keep track of the times you feel very depressed, upset, nervous, or deeply worried. Explain why you think you feel the way you do. If you can't account for your feelings, say so.

Dates from _____ to _____	Describe How You Felt	Reasons or Explanations

4. Weight-tracking

To track your weight, follow this procedure:

A. Record your height without shoes in the space provided below. If you are between ages 18 and 25, check occasionally to see if you have grown a bit. (Persons under 18 should plot changing heights and weights on the appropriate charts in the chapter "Tracking and Testing the Health and Development of Children.")

B. As a basis for comparison, record your weight at age 20.

C. Record what you consider to be an "ideal" weight for you. Refer to Tables I or II on the following pages to help you arrive at this figure.

D. Weigh yourself once a month (or as often as once a week if you are dieting) and record the date and weight on the chart below.

E. Find percent overweight or underweight:

$$\frac{\text{pounds over or under}}{\text{recommended weight}} = \text{percent over or under}$$

My height is .... _____ .

My weight at age 20 was................ _____ .

I consider my ideal weight to be ... _____ .

Date	Weight	Percent Under or Overweight	Date	Weight	Percent Under or Overweight	Date	Weight	Percent Under or Overweight

TABLE I   RECOMMENDED WEIGHTS FOR MEN
(Height without shoes, weight without clothing)

Height	Small Frame	Medium Frame	Large Frame
5' 1"	109–117	115–126	123–138
5' 2"	112–120	118–130	126–141
5' 3"	115–123	121–134	129–145
5' 4"	118–126	124–138	132–149
5' 5"	121–130	128–142	135–153
5' 6"	125–134	132–146	139–158
5' 7"	129–138	136–150	143–163
5' 8"	133–142	140–155	147–168
5' 9"	137–146	144–160	151–172
5' 10"	141–150	148–165	155–176
5' 11"	145–154	152–170	160–181
6' 0"	149–158	156–175	165–186
6' 1"	153–162	160–180	170–191
6' 2"	157–166	165–185	175–196
6' 3"	161–170	170–190	179–201

TABLE II   RECOMMENDED WEIGHTS FOR WOMEN
(Height without shoes, weight without clothing)

Height	Small Frame	Medium Frame	Large Frame
4' 8"	90–96	94–105	102–117
4' 9"	92–99	96–108	104–120
4' 10"	94–102	99–111	107–123
4' 11"	97–105	102–114	110–126
5' 0"	100–108	105–117	113–129
5' 1"	103–111	108–120	116–132
5' 2"	106–114	111–124	119–136
5' 3"	109–117	114–128	123–140
5' 4"	112–121	118–133	127–144
5' 5"	116–125	122–137	131–148
5' 6"	120–129	126–141	135–152
5' 7"	124–133	130–145	139–156
5' 8"	128–138	134–149	143–161
5' 9"	132–142	138–153	147–166
5' 10"	136–146	142–157	151–171
5' 11"	140–150	146–161	155–176
6' 0"	144–154	150–165	159–181

Narrow shoulders and pelvis = small frame; wide shoulders and pelvis = large frame

5. Occupational Health Hazards

List any possible health hazards you may be exposed to at work now, or which you may have been exposed to in the past. Include anything you may just be suspicious of, even though the substance or condition has not yet been proven dangerous, and even if employers assure you all is well. Substances once thought harmless have later been shown to be highly toxic and with long-lasting effects.

Possible occupational health hazards include:

- X rays, atomic radiation, other radioactive materials
- Any chemical you come into contact with, or fumes that you breathe. Ask about any pervasive odor that exists where you work. Try to find out what causes the odor. List these on the chart.
- Microwave radiation from ovens or transmitters
- Persistent loud noise
- Dust particles in the air—coal dust, cotton dust, dirt particles, flour, asbestos, etc.

Substance	Dates of Exposure _____ to _____	Place of Employment and Circumstances

6. Record of Physical Examinations by a Physician

List general physical examinations by a physician and note any irregularities brought to your attention as a result.

Date	Physician's name and Address	Results and Comments

7. Personal Illness Record

On the following chart itemize any important illnesses or difficulties you have had. Include childhood diseases. Record new illnesses and problems as they occur. Make a cross-record of each entry here in the health history section relating to the appropriate body system—heart and lungs, vision, skin, etc.

Enter dates, treatments received, results and how the difficulty affects you now.

Dates from _____ to _____	Illness or Difficulty	Treatment, Results, Comments

8. Operations

List any surgical operations you have had—tonsils, appendix, gallbladder, stomach, small intestine, large intestine (colon), kidney, thyroid, hernia (rupture), breast, uterus, ovaries, prostate, and any other. Tell when and where the operation was performed and comment briefly on the results.

Date	Operation	Physician and Hospital	Results and Comments

9. X ray Record

List any X rays or X ray treatments you have had, other than dental X rays. Include X rays of the chest, spine, arms, legs, stomach, kidney, intestines, gallbladder, and so on. Enter the name and address of the physician, hospital, or clinic where the X rays are on file, and briefly describe the findings.

Date	Kind of X ray	Physician and/or Hospital	Results and Comments

10. Tracking the Function of the Heart, Lungs, and Circulation

A. In the space provided below make a record of any problems you have, or have had, with your heart, your breathing, or your circulation. Include any history of high blood pressure, pneumonia or bronchitis, problems with veins or arteries, etc. Describe any treatments you have had for the problems you list.

Date	Problem	Treatment and Comments

B. The following charts provide space to record and track data relating to various aspects of the heart, lungs, and circulatory system. Detailed instructions for measuring and tracking each of these functions can be found in the chapter "Testing the Heart, Lungs, and Circulation."

PULSE

Date	Resting Pulse	Pulse after Step Test	Comments

BLOOD PRESSURE

Date	Blood Pressure Systolic/Diastolic	Date	Blood Pressure Systolic/Diastolic

RESPIRATION RATE

Date	Respiration rate	Date	Respiration rate

MATCH TEST

Date	Pass	Fail	Date	Pass	Fail	Date	Pass	Fail

VITAL CAPACITY

Indicate date and whether test was done with a spirometer or homemade equipment. Describe results.

Date	Type of test	Results	Date	Type of test	Results

11. Tracking Vision

A. Describe briefly how you use your eyes at work and at leisure. For example, a lathe operator may use his eyes at one distance most of the time, whereas a teacher may constantly shift from book, to blackboard, to the back of the classroom.

_____

_____

_____

B. Make a record of any problems you have, or have had, with your eyes. Describe any treatments you have had for the problems you list.

_____

_____

_____

_____

C. Describe results of professional eye examinations. Record eye-glass prescription, if any.

Date	Eye Doctor	Results

_____

_____

_____

_____

_____

D. The following charts track various aspects of visual function which you should check on a regular basis. In each case, the necessary data can be obtained through self-testing by carefully following the procedures described in the chapter "Testing Vision."

VISUAL ACUITY

Date	Distance Vision Without Glasses		Distance Vision W/glasses if Needed	
	Left Eye	Right Eye	Left Eye	Right Eye
	20/	20/	20/	20/
	20/	20/	20/	20/
	20/	20/	20/	20/
	20/	20/	20/	20/
	20/	20/	20/	20/
	20/	20/	20/	20/
	20/	20/	20/	20/
	20/	20/	20/	20/
	20/	20/	20/	20/
	20/	20/	20/	20/
	20/	20/	20/	20/
	20/	20/	20/	20/
	20/	20/	20/	20/
	20/	20/	20/	20/
	20/	20/	20/	20/
	20/	20/	20/	20/

NEAR POINT OF ACCOMMODATION

Date	Near Point Without Glasses	Near Point With Glasses		Date	Near Point Without Glasses	Near Point With Glasses

VISUAL FIELD

At the end of each line in the diagrams below, record the distance in inches from the dot on the wall to the point on the wall where your eye first discerns movement, as described in the test "Tracking Your Visual Field" in the chapter "Testing Vision."

Left Eye	Right Eye	Left Eye	Right Eye

Date _____
Distance from eye to
Wall _____ (inches)

Date _____
Distance from eye to
Wall _____ (inches)

| Left Eye | Right Eye | Left Eye | Right Eye |

Date _____
Distance from eye to
Wall _____ (inches)

Date _____
Distance from eye to
Wall _____ (inches)

| Left Eye | Right Eye | Left Eye | Right Eye |

Date _____
Distance from eye to
Wall _____ (inches)

Date _____
Distance from eye to
Wall _____ (inches)

| Left Eye | Right Eye | Left Eye | Right Eye |

Date _____
Distance from eye to
Wall _____ (inches)

Date _____
Distance from eye to
Wall _____ (inches)

BLIND SPOT

Following the procedure described in the chapter "Testing Vision," map your blind spot for each eye. Repeat this test every six months. Staple or clip the maps you have made to this page. On each map record the date of the test and all measurements that show how you set up the test. Be sure you duplicate the conditions of each test exactly on subsequent trials; otherwise your comparisons will be inaccurate. Comment on any changes you notice from one test to the next.

12. Tracking the Nervous System

A. Make a record of any problems you have, or have had, which a physician has said are related to your nervous system. Describe any treatments you have had for the problems you list

Date	Problem	Treatment and Comments

B. After performing the series of neurological tests described in the chapter "Testing the Nervous System," note any findings that strike you as suspicious or questionable and enter them in the chart below.

Date	Test	Comments

13. Tracking Urine and the Urinary System

A. Describe any problems you have, or have had, with your urinary system. Tell about any treatments you have had for the problems you list.

Date	Difficulty	Treatment and Comments

B. Describe any urine abnormalities* now or in the past; blood in the urine, sugar in urine, ketones, acidity, protein (albumin), bacteria, bile products, and so on. Tell how you know about them—professional evaluation or self-testing—and any treatments prescribed for the condition.

Date	Problem	How Tested	Treatment and Comments

*A discussion of urine abnormalities and self-testing procedures is presented in the chapter "Testing Urine and the Urinary System."

C. Twenty-four Hour Fluid Intake-Output Record*

Date	Amount of liquid drunk	Amount of urine passed	Date	Amount of liquid drunk	Amount of urine passed

*A discussion of urine abnormalities and self-testing procedures is presented in the chapter "Testing Urine and the Urinary System."

14. Tracking Digestive Function

A. Make a record of any problems you have, or have had, with your digestive system. Tell if these conditions were self-diagnosed or diagnosed by a physician. Describe any treatments you have had for these problems including self-treatment with over-the-counter medicines and devices (antacids, suppositories, laxatives, etc.)

Date	Problem and Location	Treatment and Comments

B. List any drugs and medicines you take for your digestive system. Include both prescription and over-the-counter medications such as antacid tablets.

Dates from to	Kind of Medication	Prescribed by doctor Yes No		Purpose

C. Use a tape measure to measure the distance around your abdomen in two places: just below the breastbone and just above the highest points on your hip bones. Recheck every six months. (Women should not check just prior to a menstrual period.)

Date	Girth Below Breastbone	Girth Above Hip Bones	Date	Girth Below Breastbone	Girth Above Hip Bones

D. Tracking problems with bowel movements and digestive upset.

Date and Time	Problem	Foods Eaten	Drugs used	Stress or Emotional Upset

15. Problems with Bones, Joints, and Muscles

A. Make a record of any problems you have, or have had, with your bones, joints, or muscles. Describe any treatments you have had for the problems you list, or what you do for the condition if you treat it yourself. Indicate if you use any braces or artificial limbs.

Date	Problem	Treatment and Comments

B. If you suspect a muscle is losing size or strength, check with a doctor and then periodically measure strength and girth of corresponding muscles according to the procedures described in the chapter "Tests and Observations of Bones, Muscles, and Joints."

Date	Location of Muscle	Measurements Left Side Right Side	Results of Comparative Strength Tests

16. Checking the Ears, Nose, Mouth, and Throat

A. Make a record of any problems you have, or have had, with your ears, nose, mouth, and throat (except dental problems). Describe any treatments you have had for the problems you list.

Date	Problem	Treatment and Comments

B. Have you ever been told you have a punctured eardrum? _____ If yes, explain the circumstances.

_____

_____

_____

C. Do you wear a hearing aid? _____ If yes, what kind? _____

_____

D. Test your hearing once a year using one of the methods described in the chapter "Testing the Ears, Nose, Mouth, and
Throat," or have it done professionally. Record the date, testing
method, and results below.

Date	Testing Method	Results	Date	Testing Method	Results

17. Dental Record

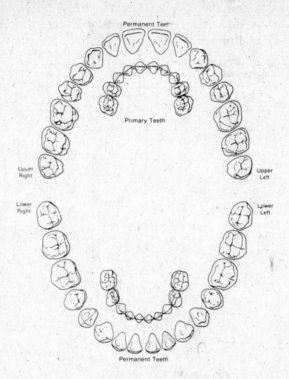

Permanent Teeth

Primary Teeth

Upper Right

Upper Left

Lower Right

Lower Left

Permanent Teeth

A. Describe any problems you have, or have had, with your teeth or gums. Since it is difficult to recall all the dental work you have had, ask your dentist to help you review by pointing out major fillings, root-canal work, crowns, missing teeth, and so on. Or, inspect yourself using the procedure described in the chapter "Testing the Ears, Nose, Mouth, and Throat." Indicate your findings on the chart above. Then start a record of all subsequent dental work. If you are not sure what the dentist is doing, ask.

Date	Work Done	Which Tooth?	Comments

B. Do you wear dentures or a bridge? _____ If yes, describe it
(whole or partial, teeth replaced).

_____

_____

_____

C. Record dates of dental self-examinations and note questions you
   want to ask the dentist. For example, you may notice bleeding
   gums, foul mouth odor when using dental floss, suspected
   cavities, sensitive teeth, etc.

Date	Comments	Date	Comments

18. Watching Your Skin

A. Make a record of any problems you have, or have had, with your skin. Describe any treatments you have had for the conditions you list. Include self-treatments as well as treatments prescribed by a physician.

Date	Problem	Treatment and Comments

B. Describe your exposure to the sun—is it a lot, a little, or a moderate amount?

	At Work	Recreation	Sunbathing	Ultraviolet Sunlamp
Now				
In the past				

C. Describe the kinds of irritants your skin has been exposed to now, in your daily work, occasionally (perhaps in a hobby), and in the past. List substances whether or not they actually irritate your skin. These should include liquid, solid or airborne substances such as dyes, gases, soaps, detergents, cleaners, paints and varnishes, strippers, commercial chemicals used in any treatment or process, exhaust fumes, smoke, dust particles, and so on.

Dates From ____ to ____	Substance	Degree of Exposure	Skin Reaction, if Any

D. Skin allergies: Name any substances to which your skin seems to be allergic—poison ivy, metals (including silver and gold), soaps, detergents, cosmetics, clothing, and so on.

Date	Substance	Kind of Reaction	Treatment, if Any

E. Examine your skin every six months. Measure and describe moles and other blemishes and irregularities, describe skin texture and color, cysts and tumors, and note symptoms such as itching, scaling, and rashes. Record your findings below. (For a discussion of these conditions, refer to the chapter "Identifying and Tracking Skin Blemishes and Ailments." Danger signs of skin cancer must be reported to a physician at once!)

Date	Findings and Comments

19. Problems with the Reproductive Organs

A. Make a record of any problems you have, or have had, with your reproductive organs or breasts. Describe any treatments you have had for the problems you list.

Date	Problem	Treatment and Comments

B. Birth-control methods or devices: Indicate what birth-control method(s) you use, if any, or have used in the past—pill, diaphragm, foam, IUD, rhythm, condom, sterilization (male or female), other.

Method or Device	Type or Brand Name	How Long Used? from _____ to _____

C. Record of Pap Smears

Date	Results	Date	Results	Date	Results

D. Rh compatibility with spouse (consult your doctor):
   Yes _____ ; No _____ .

E. Breast self-examination record: Following the procedure outlined in the chapter "Tests and Observations of the Reproductive Organs," examine your breasts on a regular, monthly basis. Make a record of the size and location of any lumps and hard spots and call these to the attention of your doctor.

Date	Results, Notes, and Comments

F. Ovulation Chart* (Basal Body Temperature Chart)

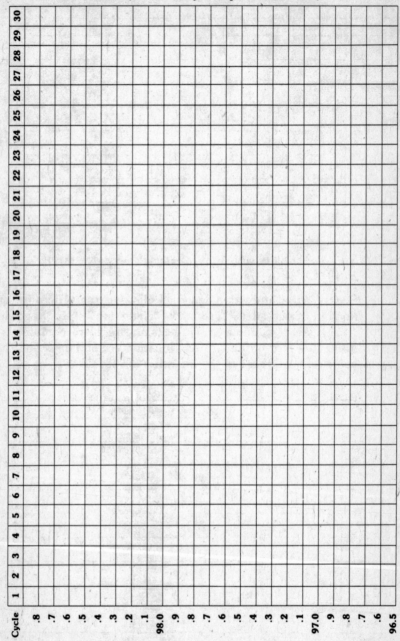

BASAL BODY TEMPERATURE CHART

*For the correct procedure to check for ovulation, refer to the chapter "Tests and Observations of the Reproductive Organs."

G. Pregnancy Records. Record all of your past pregnancies and their results. Under "Comments," describe any difficulties you had—Rh incompatibilities, birth defects, and so on.

Date	Live Births		Still Birth	Aborted	Comments
	Full Term	Premature			

H. Tracking Current Pregnancies. It is often important to know the state of your health and your health habits during pregnancy at the time of delivery, and sometimes many years later.

In the space below, keep a diary of your pregnancies. Include a record of all drugs and medicines taken (including aspirin, vitamins, and laxatives), illnesses, exposure to noxious fumes or chemicals, amounts of alcohol used, whether or not you smoke and how much, and any other information you consider interesting or noteworthy about how you carried and gave birth. Include attending physician's name and address.

Date	Events and Comments

20. Other Concerns

On this page record anything you want to comment on about your health that is not covered elsewhere. Record anything you think is important, things you will want to remember in the future, or things you think an examining doctor may want to know some day.

Date	Comments

21. A Systems Review

A *systems review* is a battery of questions designed to uncover problems you may have with one or more of your body systems. Your doctor will go through a systems review with you when you have a general physical examination, and you should do a systems review yourself about once a year between examinations.

A *"Yes"* answer to any question hints at trouble and a doctor should be consulted. If you answer *"Yes"* to a question, answer the follow-up questions as well which help to pinpoint the problem and enable you to describe the trouble more precisely to your doctor. Also refer to the chapter in the *Bodyworkbook* which applies.

Instructions: When you answer "No" to a question move immediately to the next numbered question without bothering to answer the follow-up questions.

When you answer "Yes" to a question, stop and answer the follow-up questions which apply to your problem. Add your own comments whenever you feel they are necessary or helpful.

THE NERVOUS SYSTEM

1. Have you been having headaches recently?

_____ Yes _____ No

Where are they located?

_____ Right side _____ All over
_____ Left side
_____ Front
_____ Back

Which of these describe your headache?

_____ Throbbing pain   Other _____
_____ Constant pain
_____ Tight band   _____

_____

Do any of the following occur just before or with your headache?

_____ Blurred or swirly vision _____ Nausea or
_____ Other eye trouble   vomiting
                                 _____ Stomach pains

2. Have you been having dizzy spells recently?

_____ Yes _____ No

Do any of the following apply to your dizzy spells?

_____ They occur before meals _____ I bite my tongue
_____ Eating something sweet _____ I shake all over
helps.

_____ Other (explain) _____

_____

3. Have you fainted or had a convulsion in the last year or so?

_____ Yes _____ No

_____ I fainted.
_____ I fainted *and* had a convulsion.
_____ I had a convulsion.

4. Have you noticed a paralysis or weakness in any part of your body during the past year or so?   _____ Yes_____ No

It was in my _____ and I still have it.
It was in my _____ and it went away.

_____ It started suddenly.   _____ It came on gradually.

5. Have you had any numbness or tingling in your arms or legs lately?   _____ Yes _____ No

Describe the feeling. _____

_____

Is there any special time when the feeling occurs? ____

_____

6. Have you had any problems in the following areas?

_____ Yes _____ No

_____ Speech difficulty   _____ Trembling hands
_____ Trouble with fine   _____ Memory loss
        movements such as
        writing or buttoning clothes

7. Have you been knocked unconscious in the last year?

_____ Yes _____ No

_____ I was really out cold.
_____ I was really just down and dizzy.

How did it happen?_____

_____

_____

SKIN

8. Do you have any problems with your skin, hair, or scalp?

_____ Yes _____ No

Read the following list before you decide.

_____ Unusually dry, itchy   _____ Pimples or boils
        skin   _____ Eczema
_____ Rashes or hives   _____ A nonhealing
_____ Acne   sore*
_____ Unusual reaction to   _____ A changing mole*
        sun
_____ Athlete's foot or other fungus infection

*Do not put off showing these to a physician.

16. Have you been having trouble with your throat or tonsils?

_____ Yes _____ No

_____ Throat dryness   _____ Difficulty
                                                 swallowing

_____ Frequent sore throat   _____ Tonsillitis

Other problem _____

COUGHING OR DIFFICULTY BREATHING

17. Have you been coughing a lot?   _____ Yes _____ No

The cough is
_____ worse in the morning.   _____ about the same
_____ worse afternoons and   all day and night.
              evening.

What do you cough up?
_____ Nothing   _____ Yellow-white material
_____ Green material   _____ Red or black material
_____ Frothy material

18. Have you coughed up blood in the past year?

_____ Yes _____ No

When? _____

19. Have you had difficulty breathing recently?

_____ Yes _____ No

_____ Shortness of breath   Other _____
_____ Wheezing sounds
_____ Hard to breathe   _____

_____

When does the difficulty occur?
_____ When climbing stairs   _____ When exercising
_____ All the time   _____ Seasonally (when?)
_____ Other times not   _____ When exercising
              mentioned   _____

20. Do you sometimes wake up at night because you are short of breath or you have difficulty breathing? _____ Yes _____ No

How many pillows do you use when you sleep? _____

21. Do you often wake up at night and find yourself soaked in sweat?   _____ Yes _____ No

How often has this happened? _____

_____

CHEST PAIN

22. Have you been having pains in your chest lately?
                                          _____ Yes _____ No

_____ I seem to have hurt my chest or my shoulder.
_____ It just started and I don't know why.

What is the pain like?
_____ Sharp   _____ Dull   _____ Squeezing

Where is the pain?
_____ It seems to be   _____ It seems to be
        inside.   outside around
                                             the ribs.

How bad is the pain?   _____ Not too bad
_____ Very bad
_____ Moderate

Where is the pain located, specifically?
_____ On the right   _____ In the middle
_____ On the left   _____ All over

When you feel the pain, how long does it last?
_____ A few seconds   _____ Several days
_____ A few minutes   _____ I have it most of
_____ Hours   the time.

When does the pain occur?

_____ Generally at night or in bed   _____ Mostly when I exercise

_____ Generally during the day   _____ When I'm resting

                                        _____ No special time

When you have chest pain, do you also have one or more of the following?

_____ Pain in the left arm   _____ Pain in the shoulder

_____ Pain in the jaw or neck

Do any of these make your chest pain better?

_____ Exercise   _____ Eating

_____ Medicine   _____ Rest

If medicine makes it better, what kind? _____

_____

Do any of these make your chest pain worse?

_____ Exercise   _____ Rest

_____ Food   _____ Coffee

_____ Something else _____

When you have chest pain, do you have any of these other things?

_____ Sweating   _____ Feeling of nausea

_____ Weakness   _____ I feel my heart beating.

_____ Other_____

23. Does your heart sometimes seem to beat in an unusual way?

                                        _____ Yes _____ No

_____ It beats irregularly, skips a beat.

_____ It beats very slowly.

_____ It beats very rapidly.

How often does this happen? _____

DIGESTION

24. Do you have any of the following problems with your digestion?

_____ Yes _____ No

_____ Fatty or fried foods disagree with me.

_____ These other foods disagree with me: _____

_____

_____

_____ I frequently have indigestion.

_____ My digestion is just plain bad.

25. Has your abdomen or belly gotten abnormally swollen or enlarged?

_____ Yes _____ No

How do you know? _____

26. Do you have abdominal (belly) pain, distress, or discomfort?

_____ Yes _____ No

_____ Pain   _____ Heartburn

_____ Distress   _____ Burning under the
                                                     breastbone

Something else _____

When does this discomfort occur?

_____ Before meals   _____ At night

_____ After meals   _____ During the day

Some other times _____

_____

Where would you say the pain or discomfort is located?

_____ Mostly on the left side   _____ It's all over.

_____ Mostly on the right side   _____ It spreads to my

_____ Mostly in the middle   back.

I can locate it precisely. It's _____

_____

Do you take something for your problem?
_____ Yes   _____ No
    If yes, what? (Antacid, laxative, food or drink, something
else)_____

_____

27. Have you been vomiting frequently during the past year?
                                        _____ Yes _____ No

    What does the material that comes up look like?
    _____ Like pieces of food just eaten
    _____ Like coffee grounds
    _____ Like something else (describe it)_____

_____

28. Do you have any of the following problems?
                                        _____ Yes _____ No

    _____ Frequent belching   _____ Food sticks on the
    _____ Frequent hiccups   way down.

29. During the past year, did the whites of your eyes turn yellow?
    Did your skin ever turn yellow? Were you told you had yellow
    jaundice?   _____ Yes _____ No

    _____ Whites of eyes were   _____ Skin *and* eyes
           yellow.   were yellow.
    _____ Skin was yellow.   _____ I had yellow
                                        jaundice.

30. Have you had trouble with bowel movements recently?
                                        _____ Yes _____ No

    _____ Diarrhea frequently   _____ Unable to hold
    _____ Frequently constipated   bowel movements
    _____ Pain with bowel   long enough to
           movements   get to a toilet

31. Have your stools been an unusual color or odor during the past year?

_____ Yes _____ No

_____ Black or tarlike   _____ Very light,
_____ Red or blood-smeared   almost white
_____ Unusually foul-smelling

32. Have you had any bleeding from your rectum?

_____ Yes _____ No

33. Do you think you have hemorrhoids (piles)?

_____ Yes _____ No

If yes, what makes you think so?_____

URINATION

34. Do you have any of the following problems with urination?

_____ Yes _____ No

_____ Can't always hold urine   _____ Sometimes pass
_____ Dribbling   urine when I
_____ Bed wetting   cough or sneeze
_____ Difficulty starting flow   _____ Pain or burning
                                            with urination

35. Do you often get up at night to urinate?_____ Yes _____ No
If yes, how often each night? _____

36. Have you passed red or bloody urine during the past year?

_____ Yes _____ No

37. Have you noticed any change in the force of the stream of urine during the past year? _____ Yes _____ No

38. Have you ever been told (or found by self-testing) that you have sugar or other substances in your urine?_____ Yes _____ No

If yes, what substances have been found? _____

_____

39. Do you seem always thirsty and take large quantities of fluid to relieve your thirst? _____ Yes _____ No

   If yes, have you done a fluid intake-output test (see chapter "Testing Urine and the Urinary System")?

   _____ Yes _____ No

   If you have done the test, what were the results? _____

   _____

THE REPRODUCTIVE SYSTEMS

MEN

40. Have you had any difficulties with erections recently?

   _____ Yes _____ No

   _____ It is difficult to have an erection at all. _____ Erections are often painful.

41. Have you had a sore on your genitals which did not heal properly? _____ Yes _____ No

42. Have you noticed any change in your testicles?

   _____ Yes _____ No

   _____ They seem to be getting smaller.
   _____ They seem to be getting larger.

   _____ I think a lump is developing in there.
   _____ They have become tender.

43. Do you think you are sterile (unable to father children), or do you have reason to be certain of it? _____ Yes _____ No

   _____ I've had a sterilization operation.
   _____ I have been unable to have children.

   _____ I think I'm sterile, but I'm not sure, for this reason:

   _____

_____ A physician has told me I'm sterile for this reason:

_____

44. Do you have reason to suspect you should be examined or tested for venereal disease?   _____ Yes _____ No

45. Do you think you may have prostate trouble?
    _____ Yes _____ No

    What makes you think so? _____

46. Have you developed a hernia (rupture) in the past year?
    _____ Yes _____ No

47. Have you had any swollen glands or other lumps in your groin?
    _____ Yes _____ No

WOMEN

48. Have you had a miscarriage or spontaneous abortion, or elective abortion?   _____ Yes _____ No

    _____ Attended by a physician   _____ Not attended by a
    _____ Elective abortion   physician
    _____ Miscarriage or spontaneous abortion

49. Have your periods changed during the past year?
    _____ Yes _____ No

    _____ They've become lighter.   _____ They are shorter.
    _____ They've become heavier.   _____ They always were
    _____ They are longer.   irregular but now
    _____ They are irregular.   more than usual.
    _____ Pain with periods
    _____ Bleeding between
    periods
    _____ Other change

50. Are you generally nervous or tense before your periods start?
    _____ Yes _____ No

51. Do you use any kind of birth control? _____ Yes _____ No

What kind of birth control do you use? _____

Do you have any problems related to your mode of birth control? _____

52. Have you had any unusual vaginal discharge during the past year?   _____ Yes _____ No

If yes, describe it and how long it lasted. _____

_____

53. Have you been having pain with sexual intercourse?
                                          _____ Yes _____ No

54. Do you have reason to suspect you should be examined or tested for venereal disease?   _____ Yes _____ No

BREASTS

55. Do you have any pain in your breasts? _____ Yes _____ No

56. Do you have a discharge or bleeding from the nipples?
                                          _____ Yes _____ No

57. Have you noticed a lump in either breast?
                                          _____ Yes _____ No

(See chapter "Tests and Observations of the Reproductive Organs" for a description of breast self-examination.)

58. Have you noticed that one or both of your nipples seem to be retracting into the breast?   _____ Yes _____ No

59. Does the skin of either breast seem to be puckering or dimpling?   _____ Yes _____ No

GENERAL QUESTIONS

60. Do you have any problems or complaints with your sex life?

    _____ Yes _____ No

    If yes, explain. _____

    _____

61. Have you become unusually pale recently, or do you have some reason to believe you are anemic?   _____ Yes _____ No

    If yes, tell about it. _____

    _____

62. Do you notice bruises about your body that appear without apparent reason?   _____ Yes _____ No

    Where do they occur?_____

    Do they persist or quickly disappear? _____

63. Are you generally *un*comfortable at the same temperature as most people?   _____ Yes _____ No

    _____ I'm generally hotter.   _____ I'm generally colder.

64. Are you unusually tired or sluggish a good deal of the time?

    _____ Yes _____ No

65. Do you notice any of the following occurring?

    _____ Yes _____ No

    _____ Eyes bulging, or developing a wide-eyed, pop-eyed appearance

    _____ Eating more than usual with no weight gain

    _____ A swelling in the neck

    _____ Jumpiness or unusual nervousness

66. Have you been having pains or cramps in your legs or feet?

    _____ Yes _____ No

    Where do you have the pains? _____

    When do they occur? _____

67. Have you noticed that your ankles have been swelling?

    _____ Yes _____ No

    _____ Usually swollen in the   _____ They swell only in
             evening   hot weather.
    _____ They swell only after   _____ Swollen nearly all
             I stand a long time.   the time
    _____ Other times (when?) _____

68. Have you recently developed varicose veins?

    _____ Yes _____ No

69. Do you have swollen glands or other lumps in your armpits?

    _____ Yes _____ No

70. Have your fingers or toes been getting very white frequently and easily?   _____ Yes _____ No

71. Have you had pain, stiffness, or swelling in any of your joints?

    _____ Yes _____ No

    _____ On and off
                                 _____ All the time
    Where? _____

72. Do you have any trouble with your back or neck?

    _____ Yes _____ No

    If yes, describe it. _____

    _____

    _____

73. Have any of the things listed below happened to you recently?

    _____ Yes _____ No

    _____ Tenderness or swelling   _____ Unusually stiff or
             on a bone   sore muscles
    _____ Lump or swelling
             in a muscle
    _____ Muscle seems to be getting smaller or weaker.
    Explain:_____

    _____

FEELINGS AND EMOTIONS

74. Do you often feel afraid without cause, panicky, or frightened?

    _____ Yes _____ No

75. Read the following list of statements. Do any of them apply to you? _____ Yes _____ No

    _____ My marriage is not very happy.

    _____ There is more tension at home than I can bear.

    _____ I often can't control my temper.

    _____ I'm too shy with people.

    _____ My children bother me.

    _____ I always worry about money.

    _____ Things never go right for me.

    _____ I'm just no good.

76. Are you often depressed? Do you cry easily or feel like crying much of the time? _____ Yes _____ No

77. Have you thought seriously about suicide in the past year?

    _____ Yes _____ No

INDEX